Dr Cynthia _____ erience of how incapacitating multiple sclerosis can be. She also knows what it is like to be freed again from its grip, with stick, wheelchair or scooter stored away once more. Her first very early enforced 'retirement' was broken by a return to full-time work and play! In her professional life she has taught students from over 70 different countries. Her voluntary work has included being a trustee of The Multiple Sclerosis Society, chaplaincy visiting at a local hospital, contributing to the local MS branch, counselling, writing and speaking about MS. Since her last major relapse Cynthia has had to decelerate, but recently completed a PhD in theology. She enjoys the good things of life to the full, especially the arts, travelling and messing about on the river. Cynthia is married to Karl and they love living by the Thames.

Professor Richard Reynolds has spent most of his scientific career trying to understand how the nervous system repairs itself following the damage caused by MS and how this can be boosted. Having qualified with a doctorate in Pharmacology, he has a particular interest in the development of new therapies that stop the damage to the nervous system. This work has led him to teaching both science and medical students about MS, and travelling around the British Isles to help people with the disease understand what is happening to them. At home he enjoys cooking, relaxing with his family, playing the guitar and travelling. Richard is married to Jane, has four children and lives in the Chilterns.

Coping with
Multiple
Sclerosis

A Practical Guide to
Understanding and Living with MS

Dr Cynthia Benz
& Professor Richard Reynolds

Illustrated by Shaun Williams

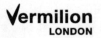

Vermilion
LONDON

5 7 9 10 8 6

First published by Macdonald Optima in 1988
Published by Vermilion in 1996

This revised and updated edition published in the United Kingdom in 2005 by Vermilion, an imprint of Ebury Publishing
Random House UK Ltd.
Random House
20 Vauxhall Bridge Road
London SW1V 2SA

The Random House Group Limited Reg. No 954009

Addresses for companies within the Random House Group can be found at: www.rbooks.co.uk

A CIP catalogue record for this book is available from the British Library

The Random House Group Limited supports The Forest Stewardship Council (FSC), the leading international forest certification organisation. All our titles that are printed on Greenpeace approved FSC certified paper carry the FSC logo. Our paper procurement policy can be found at www.rbooks.co.uk/environment

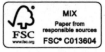

Printed and bound in Great Britain by
CPI Antony Rowe, Chippenham, Wiltshire

ISBN 9780091902469

Typeset by Palimpsest Book Production Limited, Polmont, Stirlingshire

DEDICATED

most warmly to
you
whose living is challenged by having MS.

We hope you find this book informative and encouraging
as you discover your own ways to cope with the disease.
May you live well.

ACKNOWLEDGEMENTS

We wish to express our gratitude and thanks to
MS nurses Sheila Manley and Victoria Gutteridge,
Physiotherapists Penny Dyer and Jenny Stealey
and
Consultant Neurologists Dr Omar Malak and Dr Eli Silber,
for their interest, support and kindness.
A sincere thank you to
caring friends,
and many readers, who urged for a new edition,
particularly those at the MS Stuart Resource Centre in Aberdeen.

Special appreciation and love go to
Jane Reynolds and Karl Benz
for standing by us through another time-consuming project.

Contents

ONE

What is Multiple Sclerosis?

A personal definition of MS

Anyone who has ever come into contact with multiple sclerosis will already have his or her own definition of it. Its behaviour is so infuriatingly unpredictable that no two cases are ever quite alike. Its hallmark is uncertainty – it is difficult to be certain where it begins and ends. It is as if there were on offer a kaleidoscope of symptoms, each of which comes in a variety of colours and intensities. Against that is a time factor in which symptoms appear, disappear and reappear like the most intricate movements of a bizarre dance that you have never seen before, the patterns and rhythms of which you are just getting used to when it changes totally to a haphazard jumble. MS is not easy to define simply; it revels in being elusive and difficult to catch hold of.

It helps to learn what MS can be like and what to expect. The more information you have about it, the easier it is to understand and accept. It is also important to be clear about what MS is not. It has nothing at all to do with mental disorders or so-called nervous breakdowns. It is not something you can catch like an infection. Nor is it strictly hereditary – there is no clear pattern of inheritance – although recent research does indicate that, as in the development of other diseases, one factor appears to be a genetic susceptibility towards MS. Your personal definition of MS must take account of these facts.

If you have multiple sclerosis, you have the right to your own definition of it, and the right to keep that definition open, changing it as you need to. You will meet many people who are sure they know what MS is. They may try to convince you that you are typical, atypical, better or worse off than the standard, average person with MS – they seem to know so much about it. You have the right to be yourself and to experience your MS your way.

A medical and biological definition of MS

Multiple sclerosis is an inflammatory demyelinating condition that affects the central nervous system (CNS), which is the brain and spinal cord. It is the commonest cause of neurological disability in young adults (usually defined as 18–40 years of age) in the Western world. As with many devastating and complex conditions affecting the nervous system, including Parkinson's disease and Alzheimer's disease, the initial cause of MS is still unknown. Discovering the secrets behind this complicated and unpredictable condition is like putting together a giant four-dimensional jigsaw puzzle with thousands of scientific and clinical researchers, experts in every branch of biological and medical science, painstakingly putting together the pieces they recognize and trying to add in new pieces that may or may not belong to the puzzle.

What is known about MS is that cells of the immune system, which are present in our bodies to protect against and fight off infection, enter into the CNS in large numbers, something that they do not normally do. This is known as *inflammation*. The immune cells then damage and destroy a substance called *myelin*, a fatty sheath that insulates the nerve fibres, in a process known as *demyelination*. The insulating layer of myelin around the nerve fibre allows the electrical signals passing to, from and within the brain to travel at a much faster rate. Therefore, loss of the myelin will inevitably slow down or stop the essential electrical signals. In addition to damaging the myelin, the immune cells can also damage the *axons* or nerve fibres themselves: this is called *axonal loss*. The disruption of the electrical signals within the nervous system is responsible for the wide variety of MS symptoms. The areas of myelin damage, usually referred to as *plaques* or *lesions*, are seen as scars on the nervous tissue, a process known as *sclerosis*. Since this gives rise to many areas of sclerosis in the brain and spinal cord, the disease has been given the name *multiple sclerosis*, literally 'many scars'. MS was formerly known as disseminated sclerosis because the sclerosis was scattered in the CNS.

It is easy enough to understand how an attack on the myelin sheath and the resulting damage are likely to interrupt the smooth and steady flow of impulses if you compare it with what would happen in a telephone exchange if a family of mice got in and started nibbling the insulating material around the wires. Some wires would short-circuit, leading to some telephone calls going to the wrong place or several different places, and some messages would not get through at all. In the CNS affected by MS it is demyelination that causes either distortion or blocking of messages. Either they are never transmitted to their target in the first place, they go astray completely, or they are modified or slowed down en route. MS symptoms are the visible signs of what happens to the body's functions when this occurs.

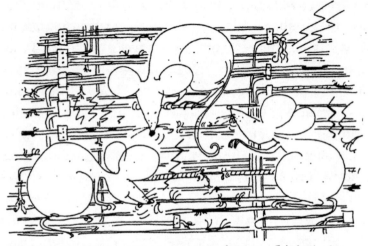

. THE EFFECT OF AN ATTACK ON THE MYELIN SHEATH CAN BE COMPARED TO THAT OF MICE NIBBLING AT THE INSULATION AROUND WIRES IN A TELEPHONE EXCHANGE ...

How does the nervous system work and how does MS change it?

The nervous system is made up of three parts: the central nervous system (CNS), the peripheral nervous system (PNS), and the autonomic nervous system (ANS). In order to understand how MS affects bodily functions it is necessary to describe the role of each of these systems.

The central nervous system is one part of the body we tend to take for granted. It operates as the body's nerve control centre and consists of the brain, the spinal cord running down the length of the backbone, and the optic nerves. The CNS links up with the peripheral nervous system. The PNS consists of all the nerves that run to and from the brain and spinal cord, linking up with our muscles, skin and joints. Information is fed back via the PNS to the CNS from muscles and sensory organs, and these electrical signals control coordination, and all movements, voluntary and involuntary. Each time you pick up a cup, play a musical instrument or drive a vehicle you are dependent on the smooth functioning of the PNS and CNS to be able to carry out such complex and skilled operations. The autonomic nervous system looks after all those bodily functions that we do not have much voluntary control over, such as the heart rate, blood pressure, sweating and the urge to pass urine. The ANS is pre-programmed and controlled by the brain, but we can exert some degree of voluntary control over some of these functions. Thus the CNS, PNS and ANS make up the nervous system, and normally these three systems work seamlessly together.

The damage caused by the immune cells in MS occurs only in the brain, spinal cord and optic nerves that make up the CNS. However, because messages to and from the body to the brain need to use the nerves of the PNS and ANS to get to their destination, and because the brain is the control centre for all of the nervous system, it seems as if MS affects the entire system. Because the electrical messages in nerves travel at very high speeds, you experience the transmission of the messages as instantaneous. It is a highly efficient body system that never takes a break, even when you are asleep. So if, owing to demyelination, there is some blockage or interference in any part of the nerve pathway that the brain is trying to use to carry out a particular body function, this may be experienced as an MS symptom.

In order to understand how MS affects the passage of these rapid electrical impulses, however simply, it helps to know something about the way nerve cells normally function. The nerve cell, or neurone, billions of which together form what we know as 'grey matter' in the brain, is the basic unit of the CNS, and is like a small computer processor. Each nerve cell has a nerve fibre, or *axon*, leading from it. Axons are like individual wires, making connections with other nerve cells, with muscles and sensory organs, such as the ears, eyes and skin, and with internal organs, such as the heart or stomach. They are fine and delicate, and can be very long – as in the spinal cord – or short, as in the brain, where compactness is crucial. When an electrical impulse has passed rapidly down the axon to reach the next neurone or to the muscle or sensory cell, it communicates by releasing a chemical called a transmitter. The chemical crosses a small gap to the next cell, which then produces its own electrical signal. It is important to understand that when our brain decides to send a message it may involve hundreds or thousands of nerve cells communicating with each other, or, in the case of a quick reflex action, such as pulling your hand away from a hot surface, it may involve only several nerve cells. It all depends on the complexity of the task that the body is trying to perform.

The role of the axons in transmitting messages is so vital that they are protected by multiple layers of a fat-rich substance called the *myelin sheath,* which is made by specialized cells in the CNS called *oligodendrocytes.* The processes, or arms, of oligodendrocytes wrap them-selves many times around the axons to produce this coating. Myelin is made up of lipids and proteins in a complex chemical substance that both protects and insulates by stopping electrical signals leaking out. Stopping the leakage also greatly speeds up their passage. Because of its colour, myelin is sometimes referred to as the 'white matter' of the brain and spinal cord. Both the oligodendrocytes and neurones are supported in their roles by other cells called *astrocytes* (so called because of their star-like shape), which help them grow and function by providing nutrients and removing other substances.

How is the immune system involved in MS?

Inflammation in the CNS and damage to the myelin sheath (demyelination) are the main causes of neurological symptoms during the early years of MS. The fine details of how the damage occurs are not certain, but it is thought to result from healthy tissue being damaged by the immune system. Since the CNS is the most vital control module in the body, any damage to it has serious conse-quences. In fact, the CNS has a unique and specialized system of protection to safeguard its function. This is called the *blood-brain barrier*, and it works as a sort of filter, keeping a close check on what substances enter the CNS. The blood-brain barrier works in conjunction with the body's own immune system, which exists to protect the body against attack by viruses, bacteria or other foreign material. The brain and spinal cord have additional

7

protection in the form of *cerebrospinal* fluid (CSF). This bathes the nerve tissue to provide a cushion, and is also thought to supply and remove chemicals and proteins to ensure balanced function. Analysis of CSF using samples obtained by a lumbar puncture may point to an unbalanced nervous system and can be used to assist MS diagnosis.

The immune system and the unique protective systems of the CNS are on stand-by in case of attack. The CNS has specialized cells called *microglia*, which carry out a constant surveillance operation to make sure that all is well. Small numbers of immune cells also move through the tissue, checking for the presence of infection, and the cross-talk between the microglia and the immune cells ensures that an immune response can be started if infection is detected. Exactly how the immune system works is not completely understood. However, what is known is that via a complex process it identifies foreign materials, viruses, bacteria and antigens, and destroys them. Normally, the immune system is able to differentiate between healthy body tissue (*self*) and invaders (*non-self*). However, with MS it is thought that the immune system behaves abnormally and attacks healthy tissue. That is why MS is described as predominantly an *auto-immune disease*. The target of the immune attack appears to be the myelin sheath and the oligodendrocyte. Whenever the immune system mounts an attack against something that it thinks is foreign, it does so by looking for particular components of invading cells, such as proteins or other chemicals. The exact components of the myelin sheath and oligodendrocyte that are recognized by the immune system as foreign are not known, and may even be different among individuals with MS. Once the immune attack has begun, the body responds by increasing its production of white blood cells (*lymphocytes*), which come flooding across the blood-brain barrier, and there is a concurrent increase in fluid, or *oedema*. The oedema itself, and the presence of large numbers of immune cells all releasing chemicals that are designed to fight off an infection, have a direct effect on the axons, and can temporarily stop the passage of electrical signals. The immune cells then begin to attack and remove the myelin sheaths, causing further disturbances of the electrical signals. Thus, in MS, the tireless protector that is the immune system changes character completely and runs amok, hell-bent on destruction.

No one can be certain what causes the immune system to begin attacking myelin in the first place, but it seems likely to be a combination of several factors. One theory is that a viral agent may play a key role in the development of MS. The virus might already be lying dormant in the body and be activated to trouble the immune system. Alternatively, by some indirect means, the virus might set off the auto-immune process. Although there is no evidence of a specific MS virus, a common virus, such as measles or herpes, could possibly trigger the auto-immune process. MS might then develop if the person is unable to shut off that auto-immune process. Whatever the trigger, it activates the lymphocytes in the bloodstream and they get through the blood-brain barrier into the brain. There they apparently join forces with other elements of the immune system to attack and destroy myelin. In response to the damage, lesions are formed at the point of attack. The areas of lesion show up clearly on magnetic resonance imaging (MRI) scans.

Some time after the attack begins and the damage is done, the inflammation dies down. Presumably at this point the immune system has been dampened down and returns to its normal state of carrying out its surveillance operation. It is likely that the body's ability to dampen down the immune system varies between individuals, and this also contributes to the variability of MS from one person to another. The myelin that was destroyed by the immune cells will now either be replaced or will remain missing. As myelinated axons can transmit nerve impulses up to ten times faster than unmyelinated axons, the body's ability to grow new myelin sheaths around the axons will contribute to the recovery from the symptoms caused by myelin loss.

If the inflammation that occurs in the nervous system was shut down once and for all after the first attack, MS would not be diagnosed, and the person would return to full health. However, we know that in the majority of MS cases the inflammation comes back again and again after variable intervals. When it comes back it does so either in the same place or at a new site or sites in the CNS. What causes the inflammation to return and why it occurs in different discrete places rather than spread all across the nervous system remains a mystery.

At this point we should return to the analogy of a telephone exchange. It is not enough just to scare off the mice nibbling at the wires and then replace the insulation: it is equally important to stop the mice returning to have another go. After a while the telephone exchange will become a patchwork of repaired and unrepaired wires that will never work as well as the original system.

Does the nervous system repair itself after MS?

If we had asked this question over a decade ago, the answer would have been that it does to a very limited extent, but not very well. Researchers have now revealed a different picture, a new part of the jigsaw puzzle. It turns out that the nervous system is usually very good at repairing damage to myelin by growing new myelin sheaths. During the early stages of MS, and possibly even later on, there is evidence that extensive repair occurs as long as the inflammation that causes the damage can be turned off. This repair can even occur after repeated damage. The extent to which this important repair process occurs may vary between individuals, and this may again be responsible for the different courses that MS can follow. However, we do know that the repair fails at some point, and that this is responsible for the lesions that can still be seen on MRI scans after many years of MS. Why this repair process fails at some point, and presumably at different times in different people, remains unknown.

One of the keys to answering the question of failing repair may lie in what happens to the nerve fibres themselves when an MS attack occurs. When the mice attack the wires in the telephone exchange, it is inevitable that some of them are completely severed by the nibbling. Recent research has shown that this is the same for MS. Even during the early stages, some of the nerve fibres are destroyed by the inflammation that causes the demyelination. They are, if you like, 'caught in the crossfire', even though they are not directly attacked by immune cells.

Fortunately, many are preserved, even though their myelin sheaths are now missing. In a telephone exchange it is possible simply to put in new wires to replace the lost ones. The central nervous system, however, does not appear to have the ability to replace lost nerve fibres, but overcomes this situation by having a lot of spare capacity. A large number of nerve fibres go to the same places to carry out the same function, so the loss of some of them does not result in symptoms. Only when the increasing loss of nerve fibres reaches a certain threshold, after which the nervous system cannot compensate for the loss, do symptoms resulting from the lost fibres become apparent. Thus we can build up a picture of an increasing loss of nerve fibres arising from repeated immune attacks at any one place. Repeated attacks will also eventually stop the repair processes that, given half a chance, would replace the myelin sheaths on damaged nerve fibres. It is this increasing loss of nerve fibres that is thought to be responsible for the long-term symptoms of MS that do not go away.

Each sclerosis or lesion has the potential to interfere with the transmission of electrical impulses along the nerve pathways that pass through that lesion. It is possible that a single lesion can cause symptoms of MS, especially if the extent of the damage to the myelin and axons is great and/or if the pathway that is damaged performs an absolutely crucial function, such as sight. However, a diagnosis of MS can be made only when a doctor is convinced that there is evidence of multiple scarring of tissue, and that is only when he or she can pick out recurring symptoms from different parts of the CNS over a period of time. Not all lesions produce obvious symptoms, however. Detailed scans sometimes reveal surprisingly large areas of sclerosis even though there have been no symptoms evident. On the other hand, just a few lesions in a couple of key places can cause a lot of havoc.

Research is being conducted and coordinated worldwide to find out the cause of MS, and how to combat the damage it does to the nervous system. Researchers are investigating the detailed mechanics of the body's immune reactions, viral attack, the metabolic system, why genetic make-up could render individuals more susceptible to MS, the effects of trauma and stress, how the repair processes in the brain work, and various combinations of these. Their discoveries help towards a better understanding of MS, an improved control of the disease and its eventual cure.

Who gets MS?

If the cause of MS were known and its course fully understood, it would be possible to predict who would be likely targets of the disease. Despite evidence from genetic studies of numerous people with MS across several continents that it is possible to be genetically susceptible to MS, it is not yet possible to test for susceptibility using simple blood analysis. However, finding out that someone may be susceptible to developing MS is very different from saying that they are likely to develop it.

Nevertheless, research throws up some interesting data that reveal certain patterns. Unfortunately, MS is a young person's disease. Its symptoms most often appear for the first time between the late teenage years and the early forties, with a peak between 29 and 33 years, although a small percentage of cases do occur even earlier (in some cases as early as 10 years). The older you get, the smaller the risk of developing MS, although in rare cases it is still possible to develop it well into the sixties.

In the most recent surveys MS was found to be twice as common in women as in men in all ethnic groups, something also known to occur in other diseases that are thought to involve an auto-immune process. Although this is the general rule, cases that start later in life are commoner among men.

The occurrence of MS varies greatly between individual countries. Generally, the closer to the equator, the fewer cases of MS there are. The temperate latitudes between 40 and 60 degrees are the high-risk zones. In the northern hemisphere this includes the British Isles, northern and central Europe, Iceland, Canada and the northern states of the USA. In the southern hemisphere New Zealand, Tasmania and the southern tracts of Australia are included. However, there are some exceptions to this trend. The incidence of MS is high in some unexpected areas, such as Sardinia and Sicily, so the distribution of MS cannot be explained on the basis of genetic and cultural history alone. Children brought up in a high-risk area who later migrate as adults to a low-risk area appear to carry with them a high susceptibility to the disease. The reverse is also true. If children have spent their early lives (pre-puberty) in a low-risk area, they do not normally develop the disease. MS is definitely more common in white races than in other racial groups. It is unknown among pure-bred Bantus and Inuit, and among Native Americans too. MS is also less common among the Chinese and Japanese, who develop a specialized sub-type of the disease.

As an example of a high-risk zone, as a whole the British Isles has an estimated one person in 650 suffering from MS. That figure, however, varies from place to place. In the south of England it is one in 1000, but it more than doubles to one in 400 in the Orkney Islands off the coast of northern Scotland, the highest prevalence in the world. Researchers are often struck by clusters of people with MS living in close proximity to each other, but the only explanations given for this have been statistical coincidence and the possibility that a high incidence of MS may reflect a specific susceptibility of the native population.

Can MS be inherited?

One of the most frequently asked questions is: once MS is in the family, can it be passed on? This very real fear needs to be talked about openly. MS is not infectious or contagious. You cannot catch it from someone else. Nor is it inherited in the usual sense of the word. However, there is evidence to suggest a genetically determined tendency that increases susceptibility to MS. Some very large studies looking at the genetic make-up of people with MS, and especially at families that have more than one member with the disease, have now been carried out across both Europe and North America. About 15 per cent of those with MS have a blood relative with it (parent, brother, sister or child). MS in parents and children is less common than MS in brothers and sisters. Studies of identical twins show that there is a significantly increased chance of developing MS than between other brothers and sisters – as high as 35 per cent. The risk of developing MS is also higher (20 per cent) in children of parents who both have MS compared with children of couples where only one parent has MS (2 per cent). Despite these figures suggesting a genetic link in families, there is no evidence that inheritance of a single gene can cause MS. It appears to be a true *polygenic disease*. This means that there are multiple genes that increase the susceptibility to MS. Each gene acts independently and exerts a small contributory effect. When all these genes are present in a family there will probably be more than one person in that family over a number of generations who develops MS. Most of these genes are likely to be involved in some way in controlling the immune response. But something else needs to happen to trigger the MS in people who are susceptible to it.

Is there an MS personality? Any answer to that is likely to be subjective, but it is tempting to agree that there are some strong characteristics that many persons with MS seem to share. The stereotype is of an active, healthy, attractive young adult who works long, hard, unselfishly and without complaint, putting up with things rather stoically. One study has shown that a higher than average percentage of people with MS are highly qualified risk-takers and ready to ask questions. Of course, it is also likely that many of these characteristics develop as a result of living with MS.

The course and types of MS

No one knows precisely what course a particular case of MS will take. If you stand back and look at the experience of a large group of people with MS, certain patterns seem to emerge. Once you move in closer and focus on an individual, it's impossible to fit any one pattern neatly to any one person. The patterns offer general guidelines only to what is within the realm of possibility. That doesn't necessarily mean that what is currently happening to you will unfold into a fixed pattern for the future. Any variation or combination is possible. MS can stop and start, idle, accelerate, reverse, and even disappear.

However, from a neurological perspective, there are recognizable types of MS. In this section we look at how neurologists classify what they find when they examine and test patients suspected of having MS and the short-hand terminology they use not only within the medical profession, but also when explaining MS to patients. Any MS classification is simply a way of making sense of what neurologists see and their interpretation of it. The way MS affects you specifically will only become clear as you learn to live and cope with it. Like life in general, it is understood best only when you – and your doctor – look back.

For most people, MS in its early stages follows a fluctuating pattern, with ups and downs, starts and stops. It's a bit like having an internal weather system of symptoms as changeable as a spring day of sunshine and showers. MS symptoms can last for minutes or days, or linger for weeks, months or years. They vary tremendously in intensity, and appear and reappear in different combinations. Any variation is possible. This is why MS is most commonly described as a 'relapsing and remitting' disease. For some it remains that way.

However, there is no set pattern of relapses and remissions, and the variations from person to person and within the course of a lifetime are infinite. Not everyone with MS is able to identify a clear-cut distinction between relapse and remission, and some fret unnecessarily as to whether they are in one or the other; it is just as common to drag along betwixt and between. This no man's land is a lonely place to be. It feels like being isolated in a tunnel with no end in sight. Suddenly you can be out in the dazzling light again, or you may linger in a grey world. You always hope there will be an end to that tunnel. For some people the grey area, in which there is no clear pattern of relapse and remission, becomes more common the longer they have MS. Their symptoms settle in, and life becomes more even and predictable. A small percentage of people diagnosed with MS never experience relapses or remissions at all, while others at some stage stop having them. They have somewhat different types of MS, called 'progressive'.

Relapsing and remitting multiple sclerosis

Certainly the most common early pattern of the disease is that of relapse and remission, terms that need to be understood. When MS flares up because of inflammation and demyelination in the central nervous system, it is known as a *relapse*. Some people refer to it as an attack, exacerbation, or bout of MS instead. New symptoms occur, or old ones you hoped had gone for ever return. This is because a new area of inflammation and demyelination is developing, or an old one is being extended/reactivated. A relapse can be quite mild or relatively severe, and last from just a day or so to a much longer period. A relapse is rarely traced to a known cause, although it's tempting to try and blame something. It is possible that it may be triggered off by infection, stress or trauma. Many people are hardly surprised when a relapse appears after a prolonged period of overdoing things – fun as well as work. Sometimes it seems as if the flu bugs that are laying everyone else low don't come out as flu in a person with MS, but aggravate its symptoms. Some prefer to call this an exacerbation rather than a relapse, since it is a more temporary form. An old symptom will appear or become exaggerated for a time – perhaps just minutes, or as long as a few days.

A *remission* is when the MS flare-up stops. The symptoms of the relapse subside and disappear either partially or completely for weeks, months, years or decades. A remission is what every person with MS longs for. It is amazing that there is the potential in our bodies for complete reversal of even the severest and most entrenched disability. In the benign form of MS (see page 20), remission is often relatively complete even after many exacerbations, and permanent disability does not develop. Remissions are thought to occur because the inflammation that starts the damage process in the brain is finally turned off, allowing the natural repair processes of the brain to take over. The ensuing recovery can take a variable amount of time, depending on where and how extensive the damage is. It is also now thought that recovery can occur because a different part of the brain can take over the function of the damaged part, rather than repairing the damage.

The relapsing-remitting type of MS affects about 85 per cent of people with the disease – twice as many women as men. It is the type that young adults diagnosed in their teens, twenties or thirties usually experience, with double vision or visual loss, sensory symptoms, such as numbness, pins and needles, tingling, weakness and unsteadiness, and bladder disturbance being typical first symptoms. Characteristically, it has an abrupt onset, and the early stages of MS are marked by relapses – either with new symptoms, or with old ones intensified, each relapse followed by a gradual easing up of these symptoms as the inflammation in the nervous system subsides and the damage is repaired.

How often relapses will occur is impossible to state with any certainty. They essentially occur at random intervals, but one figure much quoted is an average of 1.75 relapses per year for the first five years in early relapsing-remitting MS. This drops to about one per year after that. However, it is possible either to go through quite a run of them in a couple of years or so, or to seem never to emerge fully from a relapse long enough to tell. Any frequency of relapse and remission is possible. A few people find that the initial period is usually followed by a static stage, when the pattern of relapse and remission tends to settle and symptoms stabilize. They may experience only minor exacerbations due to stress, fatigue or other factors. MS can then continue indefinitely in this long-lasting or chronic way. It may hopefully subside into remission. However, most people face a variable frequency of relapses, which tend to take their toll, so that after 10–15 years approximately half of those diagnosed with relapsing-remitting MS can expect to use some sort of walking aid.

Benign multiple sclerosis

A small percentage of people with MS – 10 per cent of those diagnosed with the relapsing-remitting type – experience it in a mild form, with minimal neurological symptoms, and suffer limited and usually transitory disability that they virtually recover from completely. MS for them starts suddenly, may be inconvenient occasionally, but is, to all intents and purposes, under control, with no permanent disability expected in the future. This is a benign form of MS, which often passes unnoticed by the outside world because it is mostly in a remission stage. For some, such a remission lasts a full lifetime, with permanent recovery after the first relapse. This is more likely to be so if the initial symptom is an attack of blurred vision (*retrobulbar neuritis*) followed by a long remission, or if the initial symptoms are sensory ones. When MS runs such a very benign course, it never really affects the activities of daily living in a major way. No one knows why it stays benign: either the initial attack is never repeated, or there is very little external evidence of demyelination. One can speculate that for these people their immune system is able to completely shut off the attack on the nervous system so that it does not recur. A few people even live long, full and active lives, with never a suspicion of MS, yet a post-mortem examination will reveal extensive areas of lesion. So in some cases MS need not disrupt the lifestyle of the individual or family, and may not turn out to be a major health problem.

Progressive types of multiple sclerosis

The benign form of MS described above is one end of the scale of the relapsing-remitting type. The general neurological rule of thumb suggests that within the first 15 years after the symptoms of demyelination become evident, the degree of disability you experience may give something of a rough guide to your future with MS. If you are only mildly affected thus far, you are likely to remain this way.

Inevitably, though, the pattern of MS you remember and recoil from most is the one that stares at you from pictures in charity appeal literature. It tugs at your heart-strings, and rightly so, for a small proportion of people with MS (around 10–20 per cent) are more severely afflicted with one of two different progressive forms.

The longer you live with relapsing-remitting MS, the greater the probability that you will eventually move into a secondary progressive stage. This later stage of MS, which follows the slow relapsing and remitting start, may affect up to about 45 per cent of people. After some years (usually 15–25) the acute episodes of MS are followed by an increasingly incomplete recovery so that a slow progression of permanent symptoms develops. There has to be evidence of slow but sustained deterioration for 6–12 months at least for a diagnosis of secondary progressive MS. It feels as if MS has wormed its way in when physical symptoms relentlessly worsen and disability more or less settles in. This seemed to be the way Charlotte's MS was going, and with a young family of three children under five, life looked short and bleak. Then there came a halt – remission brought a reprieve – and she slowly coasted along a slightly sloping plateau, but with occasional clear improvements visible. Those who knew her at her lowest were amazed at her spells of recovery against all odds. At this stage relapses commonly become less frequent, and not so obvious when they do occur; consequently remissions are less evident too. There are, of couse, exceptions either way, a fact that will not surprise those of you with MS.

Some 10 per cent of men and women in equal proportion experience progressive MS from the start, which will confine them, possibly sooner rather than later, to a wheelchair and perhaps, at a later stage, to bed. Primary progressive MS tends to start later in life, the first defining symptoms appearing from the mid-forties onwards, although there will have been evidence of symptoms before. As the spinal cord is particularly affected, the typical characteristics for 85 per cent of people diagnosed with primary progressive MS are walking problems, with weakness and stiffness in the legs, difficulties with balance, and impaired bladder, bowel and sexual function. People with primary progressive MS are usually visibly disabled because of loss of mobility and unsteadiness. Their symptoms neither relapse nor remit: there is always an incomplete recovery from damage. However, the progression can vary from being very rapid to very slow indeed.

It has often been suggested that these different patterns of MS may in fact represent different diseases, but it is generally agreed in the medical profession that they represent a broad spectrum of ways in which a single disease can affect individuals with different genetic make-ups.

What does the future hold?

Life expectancy with MS is as variable as everything else about the disease. Overall it is close to the norm, and generally at least 25 years from the onset. However, it can also be severely reduced if, as happens rarely, the course of MS becomes rapidly progressive. Should primary or secondary progressive MS ever move into an acute crisis stage fast, it can prove fatal: thankfully, this is exceptionally uncommon. If anything, life expectancy for women is statistically slightly less. However, Hilary, now in her eighties, has had MS since her early thirties. She has two sons, and, despite being in a wheelchair for over 40 years, gets out and about with the help of her caring husband. Her cheerful resilience and warmth are inspiring, as is her quality of life.

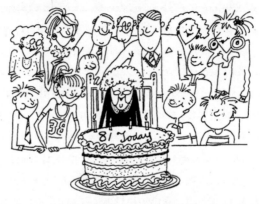

M S   IS   NOT   NECESSARILY A DISEASE YOU DIE OF.....

The relationship between the body and the emotions is very important in MS, not only in relapse and remission, but also within the fluctuations possible in MS in any given day. Mood swings are very common and perfectly understandable because with MS you never know what to expect. Just when you think you have come to terms with one way of feeling, you get catapulted to another, and adjustment starts all over again. Any damage to the brain is characterized by accompanying emotional ups and downs, and this is especially true for MS. Demyelination can have a physiological effect on the emotions, either intensifying or depressing them. It is important to accept this as fact. A person with MS will sometimes feel unreasonably or inexplicably sad, angry, fearful or happy. A later section in the book will investigate how to cope with this.

Since MS is so unpredictable, it is important to take it a day at a time, whatever pattern or stage it seems to be in. Neither you nor anyone else knows where it will take you next. It is understandable to panic at times about what can happen with MS, but you should never make assumptions about tomorrow on the evidence of today. If you can allow your panic to run its course without taking undue notice of it, you will find you come through. It is at such times that people with MS long to know how everything will turn out. They think it would help to know what pattern they fit into and what the future holds. No one can give them that information. That may be just as well, for once you fit MS too neatly into a mould, it tends to get stuck there. Christopher was permanently angry with his doctors for not being able to tell him what to expect next with MS. He came across as being aggressive, irritable, overexcited and unable to settle to living. He was so busy being upset with the unpredictability of his MS that he wasn't giving himself a chance. Do what you can gently to give your body every chance of rehabilitation whenever possible. This includes keeping your muscles supple, getting all the rest and exercise you need and want, eating a healthy diet, and keeping a positive attitude. This may seem a tall order when the going is rough, but it's one that pays dividends.

Symptoms of MS

The presence of symptoms, verified by a neurologist and backed up by brain scans, is proof of MS, and it is against these symptoms that the daily battle must be waged. As the damage that MS causes can happen anywhere in the brain and spinal cord, any bodily function can be affected at some stage, although some symptoms are rarer than others. Damage can occur not only in both the sensory and motor parts of the central nervous system, but also in areas of the brain that control thought patterns and emotions – essentially all those things that make us who we are. Therefore, symptoms can affect the sensory areas of the body: skin, muscles, joints, and particular organs, such as the eyes or ears. Motor symptoms occur when the contraction of particular muscles, anywhere in the body, does not occur properly or is not coordinated. Another group of symptoms, called 'cognitive', relate to the way that the brain processes information, which may be changed in some way by the damage that MS causes. These symptoms include memory problems, changes in mood, and reduced ability to reason and plan. Individual symptoms result from inflammation and demyelination in various parts of the brain and spinal cord, but it is clear that damage in some areas is more likely to show up as symptoms than others.

When discussing symptoms, doctors will give information about MS that may at first seem contradictory. On the one hand, they may reassure you that you are unlikely to develop many symptoms, while on the other hand, they will tell you straight that MS is a disease that cannot be controlled. If MS is uncontrollable, it should follow logically that there's nothing to stop you from developing all the symptoms going. Fortunately, that is not the experience of most people with the disease. The symptoms cover a wide range, and you certainly don't have to have them all to have MS. In fact, it is highly unlikely for any individual to experience all the possible symptoms during their life with MS.

For a diagnosis of MS to be made, neurologists must be certain that the patient has had a minimum of two attacks and that two or more areas of the central nervous system are involved. These will generally be visible as lesions on MRI scans. Symptoms must either be clearly visible during a minimum of two distinct relapses separated by an interval of several months in relapsing-remitting MS, or be obvious from clinical evidence as persistent deterioration over several months in primary progressive MS, for a definite diagnosis to be made. It is important to understand that other central nervous system diseases can share some of the same warning signs as multiple sclerosis, so some MS-type symptoms can have quite another cause. Diagnosis is discussed further in Chapter 2.

Unpredictability and fluctuation are characteristic of MS symptoms. You never know when they are going to appear or disappear, how long they will stay and how intensely they will be experienced. Symptoms are at their most troublesome during relapse, when they appear, intensify and generally make their presence felt. During remission they generally ease up, and rarely persist as strongly; often they can clear away completely. Certain symptoms hang on with grim determination, but many are transient.

Symptoms come in varying strengths. The majority are felt only in a mild way, so you may even begin to believe you are imagining them. But just as you are getting used to a certain symptom, it may vanish like a will-o'-the-wisp, and it's only then, without it around, that you are convinced it was for real. It's amazing how much one can put up with that's not normal; no wonder people with MS feel relief and an exhilarating sense of well-being when a symptom goes away. Sometimes you read about a symptom, or hear talk of one, and are surprised to discover that what had always been shrugged off as a passing inconvenience actually merits the term 'symptom'. However, it is also an inescapable fact that for some people MS symptoms can be severe, devastating and at times extremely persistent. In such circumstances it seems as if they will never ease off. Sadly, in a very small percentage of cases that is true, but normally there is some let-up. Symptoms that persist indefinitely can be really dispiriting unless some way is found of incorporating them into life, rather than constantly fretting to be rid of them.

In the light of what you have just read you may well be anxious and frightened about the symptoms that can result from the inflammation and demyelination caused by MS – quite understandably – and it is not surprising if people with MS find themselves shying away from meeting other people who are also disabled with MS; they fear that the symptoms they see may afflict them in turn. What they overlook is the fact that MS is renowned for its fluctuating range of symptoms that vary in intensity and duration. Being confined to a wheelchair in the morning doesn't inevitably mean you will still need to be in one in the afternoon.

Another understandable fear arises from the fact that symptoms seem to appear and disappear at will. If you are currently troubled by a particular symptom, the possibility that it will just go gives hope. The reverse, when you are in remission and symptom-free, is more threatening. This is a threat that will not go away, a sword of Damocles, and only the person experiencing this fear can choose whether to ignore it and get on with living, or else spend time agonizing over what could happen. Giving way to negative thinking does not help. Being positive and realistic does. It is important to keep in mind that the body is made to revert to healthy balance and fullest function. The positive set of the mind will be a vital factor in this taking place. It is also true that the central nervous system has amazing powers of healing. There is plenty of evidence from MS research that this healing process can involve the replacement of myelin (*remyelination*). There is, in fact, the very real potential for MS symptoms to disappear permanently thanks to this successful repair process.

The next section of this chapter includes a comprehensive list of symptoms, some of which are also discussed in greater detail later in the book. It is not exhaustive because the variability of MS means that there are very few neurological symptoms that have not been seen in at least a few individuals with MS. You may be relieved to find your troublesome symptom isn't unique to you but within the range of MS normality. Remember again that some symptoms can be caused by something other than MS. Sometimes it may be difficult to work out what is a symptom and what can be blamed on something else.

Having MS does not make one immune to the many other challenges that the body has to face, including normal ageing. It is very important that symptoms caused by something other than MS are treated as such.

Everyone is different in the way they cope with their symptoms. A few capitalize on very little, and take great pleasure in sharing what they have been through, often exaggerating it. It serves to get them an audience for a short time, and they feel better for having dumped the load. Others, different in personality, accept the need to talk through what it feels like having to put up with symptoms. By talking about their experience to the sort of people who will offer understanding and support, and by releasing some of the associated tensions, emotions and fears, they are able to cope. Yet others never talk about what symptoms are affecting them and just get on with it.

Invisible symptoms

These are the symptoms the person with MS is acutely aware of and discomforted by. They are the ones the non-MS person cannot see, never dreams exist, ignores or belittles, and for which only grudging sympathy is given. Sometimes they are the most troublesome of the lot. Their onset can be very rapid.

PECULIAR SENSATIONS

The most bizarre symptoms defy imagination and description. How can you explain the irritation of a trickling, twitchy feeling down a leg, hot and sweaty – or cold and clammy – feet or hands, the unrelieved heaviness of limbs? Most people have experienced pins and needles, but rarely for days at a time. Then there is a creeping numbness that often starts in the feet and works its way gradually to the waist. Impairment of touch results in a multitude of tingling sensations, many of which can be painful. Walking can be experienced as floating, trudging through water or snow, or making your way over eggs. Your whole body image can be disturbed, as if you don't know where different parts of the body are. The head feels detached, and sight feels limited to a thin slit of vision. A change in sensitivity to heat is also a recognized symptom, and this can cause a temporary worsening of other MS symptoms. Such symptoms are caused by damage occurring to the sensory pathways that bring information back to the brain from the skin, joints and muscles. These sensory pathways tell us about what is happening in our immediate environment in terms of temperature, what we are touching and also where the various parts of our

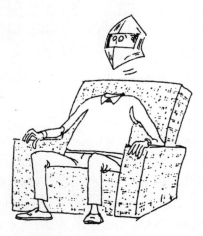

THE HEAD FEELS DETACHED FROM THE BODY AND
SIGHT FEELS LIMITED TO A VISOR OF VISION...

body are. Without these pathways working properly, we may not know the exact position of our arms or legs for example. These sensory symptoms are very common in MS, and often occur at the beginning.

FATIGUE

To relatives and close friends, fatigue can seem like a symptom of convenience – the sort of symptom you might use to escape work if you didn't have MS and weren't the sort of person who habitually saw a task through to the bitter end. Sometimes fatigue is a permanent symptom that drags around with you. At other times it creeps up unnoticed, and when it becomes apparent, it's too late. The typical pattern is to start on a project – cleaning, walking, dancing, whatever – and perform quite normally until suddenly your energy goes and you seize up or flop. The energy loss can be so immediate that you are taken quite by surprise. It is frequently accompanied by a dazed feeling and inability to communicate. Extreme weakness makes the fatigued person with MS unable to enter into arguments or work out reasons. There is a partial shut-down, and all incentive to communicate simply disappears. Some people even fall asleep. Everything, even thinking, becomes too much of an effort. Naturally, unless this symptom is understood and accepted, it has very adverse effects on relationships.

Fatigue is probably one of the few symptoms of MS that cannot be related to damage in a particular place in the nervous system. Although the cause of the fatigue remains poorly understood, it is tempting to speculate that it might arise because the nervous system is working extra hard to compensate for the MS, and repair processes are working overtime. More will be said about fatigue in Chapter 4.

VERTIGO/DIZZINESS

One of the most disturbing symptoms of MS some people experience is vertigo. It can vary from a little light-headed dizziness to a feeling that the world is turning upside-down and tipping you off it. It can also be accompanied by nausea, vomiting and an inability to walk straight and upright – or at all. The reason for this is that MS disrupts the pathways between the brain and the inner ear, which are responsible for balance, causing a loss of position-sense, and consequent problems with balance.

BLADDER PROBLEMS

The need to pass water frequently and urgently is a distressingly unwelcome symptom. It limits excursions to those where a loo is in quick reach. Although it's no joking matter, it does help if you can deal with it in a light-hearted way. On a theatre visit, Barbara was confronted with a long queue outside the ladies' loos. In desperation she shouted out that she had MS and had to get to the toilet immediately. At once doors flew open and she was able to take her pick. Her bold exclamation brought instant response and a few chuckles.

Sometimes the reverse is the problem, and urine is retained, causing uncomfortable feelings of being bloated. This is most often a problem for women rather than men.

INCONTINENCE

This is a symptom dreaded by people with MS. Like other symptoms, it can come without warning and disappear again like magic. It may be partial or total, and affect the bladder and/or bowels. Constipation may or may not accompany it.

PAIN

Many persons with MS suffer a fair amount of pain, but it is only recently that some in the medical profession have accepted the reality of that symptom. Many different types of pain can be experienced: numb aching, pins and needles, tingling sensations, sharp shooting and stabbing pains, dull, gnawing nerve pains in an arm or leg, aching eyes (like in a bad toothache), backache due to the strain of walking with difficulty, muscle spasms and cramps, with legs shooting out straight or bending sharply – most often in bed at night. The head and face can also be affected, and *trigeminal neuralgia* is sometimes experienced. This is an agonizing nerve pain in one side of the face; it lasts only a few seconds, and is accompanied by an involuntary contortion of the facial muscles that looks like a grimace.

HEARING PROBLEMS

Although deafness and tinnitus resulting from a brain-stem plaque are rare, some people with MS report impairment of their hearing. It is not so much that sounds cannot be heard, as that they don't seem to 'unscramble' sufficiently to make complete sense. This can be caused by damage to the nerves leading from the ear and by damage in the higher centres of the brain that interpret sounds.

SIGHT PROBLEMS

Although not strictly invisible symptoms, sight problems are included here because many visual difficulties are usually transitory and rarely stay long enough to be noticeable to an observer. They can, however, distress, frighten and irritate. No one likes having vision problems, but at least 70 per cent of people diagnosed with MS have to deal with sight problems at some stage. Many of these report blurred or double vision (*diplopia*), or vision with blind spots (*scotomata*) as an early symptom of MS, which normally clears up. There may also be temporary spells when there is a dimming of colour appreciation, and times when contrasts of shade are not as sharp as normal. Many of these symptoms are due to *optic neuritis* – inflammation in the optic nerve that leads from the retina to the brain – which occurs in about 20 per cent of people as one of the first symptoms of MS. Changes to the way the eyes move are also common symptoms of MS, and are caused by damage to the area of the brain that controls the eye muscles, rather than damage to the optic nerve itself. Problems with rapid eye movements, especially when scanning a page or looking from side to side, are common in MS, as are problems with moving both eyes together. A few people will experience permanent, total or partial loss of sight, with a severe loss of central vision.

SEXUAL PROBLEMS

These will be dealt with in detail later, but it is important to include them here since they can have a serious effect on relationships and cause considerable distress. Men with MS may find themselves unable to sustain an erection long enough for satisfactory intercourse. Women may experience an absence of vaginal sensation, or a distortion of it. Both men and woman may suffer from diminished arousal.

EMOTIONAL PROBLEMS

With so much going on in the body, and so many adjustments needing to be made, it is inevitable that people with MS are going to experience a wide range of emotions. There is also evidence that MS can cause magnified emotional reactions, leading to marked swings of mood. Sometimes it is impossible not to react with increased emotion, because it springs up without rhyme or reason. At other times the emotional state may be accepted as appropriate – following initial diagnosis, for instance, or after a relapse or crisis. Such symptoms can be caused by inflammation and demyelination in the area of the brain that controls emotions, but may also occur in response to the diagnosis or crisis.

MEMORY AND CONCENTRATION PROBLEMS

At times you may recognize problems to do with memory loss, and perhaps find yourself waiting for the wrong bus or entering the wrong shop. Your friends may take it lightly, but you might find it embarrassing and inconvenient. You need to accept it as a symptom of MS, and be able to recognize it when it happens. In a similar way, you may become aware of problems with concentration or reasoning, which may interfere noticeably with the sort of work you do. The medical term for these problems is 'cognitive difficulties' (see page 178).

PSYCHOLOGICAL REACTIONS

It is not uncommon to find yourself involved in a mental battle as you try to distinguish between the reality of what's going on in your body and what you fear you are imagining about yourself. Some people sidestep the truth about how fatigued they actually are and what symptoms they are having to put up with. Instead, for various reasons, they interpret them in predominantly psychological terms. This usually means that they blame themselves for what has gone wrong in their bodies. It doesn't help one jot, but it is their way of coping for the time being. It also has the effect of confusing family, friends and doctors as to what is really going on, and can thus make it harder for them to provide understanding and caring support.

Visible symptoms

These are the symptoms that everyone can see. Obviously troublesome, they also attract attention. If you are confined to a wheelchair or walk with difficulty because of MS, you are noticed. You fit the classic picture of the disease, and people react to it. Whether they smother you with attention or studiously ignore you, they cannot help but register the reality that you have MS. There is no denying visible symptoms.

And yet, despite their appearance, they need not be any more troublesome than the invisible ones. Visible symptoms fluctuate too in their duration and intensity. What is here today may indeed be gone tomorrow, or the day after.

WEAKNESS

While weakness may be limited to one or several parts of the body, it may also be an overall feeling of not having your usual amount of strength. It shows as you drag a leg, find climbing stairs a problem, or walk instead of run. It shows when you sit down to iron or peel potatoes. It shows whenever you flop into a chair or bed when you would normally have kept going. Others may not always immediately attribute it to MS, but they are clearly puzzled by this unaccustomed weakness.

To get rid of it, you might try all the common pick-me-ups, and follow advice to 'snap out of it' and 'pull yourself together'; but this is MS weakness, which is physiologically induced and can't be switched off at will.

WALKING DIFFICULTIES

For a while, you can cover up obvious stiffness as a result of over-exercise or a matter of age, but other walking problems aren't quite as easy to explain away. Lack of co-ordination, loss of balance, knees that give way so that

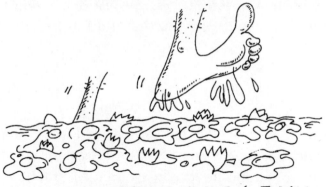

WALKING CAN BE EXPERIENCED AS FLOATING, TRUDGING
THROUGH WATER OR MAKING YOUR WAY OVER EGGS ...

you trip or topple over, the ataxic gait that resembles a
drunken stagger – these are much more difficult to
explain. Leg muscles can become weakened or paralysed.
Feet (and hands too) can suffer from cramp-like contractions. Thus, mobility can be made difficult in many ways.
Getting from one place to another becomes a strategic
operation, and you resort to using sticks, frames, scooters or wheelchairs to make getting around easier and
faster.

CLUMSINESS

The smooth, controlled movement you normally make to
carry out specific actions, such as putting on make-up,
lighting a match, or picking up a tool or piece of equipment, can become clumsy and inaccurate when you have
MS. Others notice that you drop things and have more
than your fair share of accidents. You may sometimes
suffer from wobbly movements or tremors as you try to
tackle everyday tasks. Muscle tone is altered, and can
produce spasticity or muscle stiffness, which can affect

movement. The correct messages just don't seem to be getting through to your muscles, and this is showing in how you move.

SPEECH DIFFICULTIES

If the tongue and other muscles involved in speaking are impaired, or there is damage to the areas of the brain that compose and initiate speech, a variety of problems may result. The mildest of these is a slowing down of speech, especially when tired. More seriously, and usually much later, speaking may become slurred or jerky and garbled, like a mechanical toy. Naturally this can form a barrier to communication and cause distress to everyone involved in a conversation.

CIRCULATION PROBLEMS

The effects of poor circulation can become visible, particularly with your feet, if you become very sensitive to cold and need to wrap up very warmly. It's no fun needing to wear boots or thick woollen socks with party gear. Ankles very often swell up, and you can feel quite uncomfortable.

Coping with symptoms

Whether MS affects you little by little, like fine rain that gradually soaks through to the skin, or whether it quickly clasps you in an iron grip, you cannot escape the fact that you now have to make space in your life for a chronic illness. The daily battle with the fluctuating disease

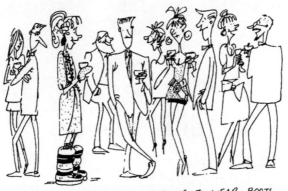

IT'S CERTAINLY NO FUN NEEDING TO WEAR BOOTS
OR WOOLLEN SOCKS WITH PARTY GEAR...

touches you at a deep psychological level. You can try to
squeeze it out, but it won't disappear, except in natural
remission. On the other hand, you can cope with it
provided you face up to the impact it will have on you,
then move on, incorporating a new dimension in your
life. Perhaps it is like the dark backcloth against which
many shades of colour really stand out. While no one can
welcome having MS, it can be turned to advantage. It
needn't be a disaster, and you can still enjoy life. We are
always struck by the countless times we've heard young
people with the disease confess that once they have got
over the initial shock of learning to live with MS, they
realize their diagnosis has given them an opportunity to
take stock. Hesitantly, for they do not see themselves as
heroic, they express a grudging gratitude that something
like MS has pushed them to re-evaluate their lives. What
psychological barriers need confronting, and how to do
so, are matters dealt with later in this book.

TWO

MS diagnosis and its consequences

Diagnosis is a pivotal point. There was life before MS, life continues after it, and the diagnosis stands starkly between. There is no one with MS who does not remain acutely aware for a long, long time, if not for ever, of when, where, how and by whom the diagnosis was or was not made clear. MS diagnosis is a loaded term, and in an uncanny way never fails to arouse a gamut of strong feelings and reactions.

Is there a right time to make a diagnosis of MS? It is devastating to be given it too soon, and infuriating to be held out on. It would take more than the wisdom of Solomon to judge the right time for everyone. But by far the majority would prefer a clear diagnosis sooner rather than later. Today it is rare for any doctor to hold on to his suspicions and simply wait for further evidence. With ongoing advances in clinical diagnosis, there is normally no need for lengthy waits, and every advantage is to be gained from beginning any available treatments as soon as possible. In any event, quite a proportion of people with MS have guessed their diagnosis first. If you are not yourself suspicious and prone to self-diagnosis, there is no doubt that your family and friends will have bombarded you with a thousand and one reasons for your condition.

Most people with MS are told their diagnosis by a doctor, normally a neurologist. A very small number discover the truth from a relative or by other means. However and whenever you receive your diagnosis you are likely to experience shock. The build-up of symptoms and all the difficulties that preceded the diagnosis take their toll in terms of stress. Learning how multiple sclerosis impacts physically, and absorbing the implications in terms of lifestyle, relationships, employment and mobility, present a huge challenge that can feel overwhelming.

Making the diagnosis

Although there is no single specific test for diagnosing MS, there are various ways in which neurologists can be confident in reaching a diagnosis. Crucial among these is locating what is going on within the central nervous system. The sclerosis, plaques or lesions responsible for damaging the myelin sheath and causing telltale symptoms cannot be seen with the naked eye. They can, however, be located in other ways, including MRI scans. This test, though, is not always necessary. Often the patient's medical history, together with a physical examination, provide sufficient information for a firm diagnosis. Other objective laboratory tests are sometimes required as confirmation. In addition, doctors will be looking for many different types of information. They will want to know when and at what age any of the symptoms became noticeable. They will be interested in where in the body symptoms have occurred, what sensations they have caused, and what effects they have had. They will need to be satisfied that two separate areas of the central nervous system have been involved. One of two patterns with regard to time should become obvious: either at least two clear-cut episodes of symptoms each lasting a reasonable period of time and separated from each other by a time gap, or the slow, progressive development of one pattern of symptoms over a long period of time. A pattern of relapse and remission may also point to a diagnosis of MS.

Typically, a patient's medical history is corroborated by the findings of a physical examination by a neurologist. Part of this examination of the central nervous system will involve testing reflex pathways; for example, by tapping the knee with a surgical hammer. Measuring how much sensation there is in response to a stimulus is done by the pin-prick and/or cotton-wool test. In addition to reflexes and sensations, checks will be made on coordination, walking, standing, grip, eye movements and the functioning of the optic nerve. With MS the neurologist will normally find some objective abnormality. In these ways he begins to build up a picture of which nerve pathways are currently affected. Illnesses other than MS that could give rise to similar symptoms must be positively eliminated first. It must be stressed that an MS diagnosis is always a clinical one based on definite criteria. It isn't a diagnosis snatched out of the air when all other likely diseases have been ruled out. Your neurologist must be satisfied that your symptoms and findings cannot be explained by anything other than MS.

Patterns of MS

Of the two basic patterns of MS, the relapsing form is predominantly inflammatory, while the non-relapsing form is degenerative. What happens within the central nervous system of a person with MS is very individual and works to no set agenda or timescale. The skill of the neurologist lies in assessing what specific damage is affecting the CNS, and if it is currently being triggered by inflammation or degeneration.

RELAPSING MS

In order to make a diagnosis of relapsing MS, a neurologist needs to be satisfied that the symptoms stem from demyelination in at least two separate areas of the central nervous system. There must be *multiple* lesions or sclerosis scattered about and affecting different parts of the CNS. In addition, the symptoms need to appear over a period of time, independently of each other and separated by a time gap. That is why it is normal practice to have a second MRI scan some time after the initial one.

The existence of symptoms is usually confirmed by internal evidence – the sclerosis, plaques or lesions in the brain or spinal cord that mark the sites of demyelination. Since lesions are good markers or indicators of MS, it is important to locate where they are and to check whether new lesions develop subsequently. Although they cannot be seen with the naked eye, lesions can be picked up using various tests, and in particular by an MRI scan.

NON-RELAPSING MS

The non-relapsing pattern of MS works differently and indicates a slow progressive development of one or more patterns of symptoms over a long period of time. This is quite a different scenario from relapsing MS. It commonly happens that patients with non-relapsing MS display less abnormality on MRI scans. They may appear visibly disabled but the lesions you would expect to see to confirm MS are simply much less frequent. Many of the lesions are described as being hidden or silent. The inflammation that highlights the lesions in relapsing MS is not present to the same extent. Degeneration has gone a stage further. The symptoms and disability result primarily from damage to the axons, which is not visible on MRI scans.

Tests to aid diagnosis

When a diagnosis of MS is strongly suspected, and supported by physical examination and clinical evaluation of your case history, you are routinely offered an MRI scan, and may also undergo other laboratory tests, as described below.

EVOKED POTENTIAL TESTS

As demyelination has the effect of slowing down the rate at which messages are transmitted along the nerve pathways, tests are done that measure how fast the central nervous system can respond to rapidly repeated stimuli.

The most common of these tests is the *visual evoked*

response (VER). You sit in front of a screen with an alternating chequer-board pattern, which evokes certain responses in the brain. Electrodes lightly glued on to your scalp record how quickly the brain responds to what the eyes see, and a computer printout records the information. It takes half an hour to have this test, and it causes no discomfort at all.

Two other tests that operate along similar lines are *brainstem auditory evoked potential* (BAEP) testing which assesses hearing, and *somatosensory evoked potential* (SEP) testing, which assesses reaction to touch.

MRI SCANS

Magnetic resonance imaging (MRI) is a computer-assisted imaging technique that exposes you to a strong magnetic field rather than X-rays, and produces 3-D images of the central nervous system. It has a remarkable sensitivity and can pick out all but the very small plaques, including those 'silent' ones not associated with any reported symptom. So detailed is the information that it is possible to see exactly what is happening to the plaques, and to measure the sclerosis so that changes can be determined in any subsequent scans. MRI can be of enormous help in diagnosis, provided it is used in conjunction with clinical information. It is also very useful in monitoring the effects of new treatments on the disease. Most clinical trials now use repeated MRI scanning to determine whether the drug being tested has any effect on the appearance of new lesions. When combined with an injection of a substance that can be viewed when it crosses the blood-brain barrier, MRI scanning can also show up very early plaque formation.

LUMBAR PUNCTURES

In a lumbar puncture a small amount of *cerebrospinal fluid* (CFS) is extracted from the vertebral column for laboratory analysis. In 90 per cent of people with MS this fluid contains antibodies – specifically, increased levels of gamma globulin and oligoclonal bands – evidence of inflammation in the central nervous system. In the early stages of MS it is rare for positive findings to show up.

Since the advent of MRI, lumbar punctures are less often used. They can cause discomfort, and some people suffer from bad headaches afterwards. It is therefore best to remain lying down immediately after the test, and especially if a headache develops. If you do get any unpleasant side effects, resting horizontally for as long as you need to is the best antidote.

ELECTROMYOGRAPHY

This is a technique used to measure how long it takes a nerve impulse to travel along the central nervous system to a muscle. It involves using an electromagnet together with electrical stimulation of the spinal cord.

Receiving the diagnosis

MS is a serious disease, and the diagnosis of it is usually a devastating blow to the patient. In an ideal world it is best to be told frankly and openly by a trusted GP or neurologist, especially if there is already a caring relationship between the doctor and patient. It takes time for the implications to sink in, and a future appointment will need to be made for you (and your partner or significant people in your life) to come back and ask all those questions that shoot right out of your mind at times of stress and shock. If possible, neurologists will involve a third professional party when they give the diagnosis, and this member of the health team will take responsibility to give care and support as needed in the future. Increasingly, this person is a specialist MS nurse, but it could also be a social worker. Either will make time available to talk over exactly what the doctor said, to answer questions and to offer support. He or she can also point out other sources of information and support, such as the national multiple sclerosis charities, the nearest branch of the MS Society, for example, or perhaps a local support group for the newly diagnosed. Whether you have the disease or live close to someone who has it, you may want to know a lot more about MS and what you can expect. It is appropriate for the doctor and his team to offer you that support, and to give the facts realistically and with optimism.

There is double pain when the diagnosis is given badly, in an off-hand and dismissive way by some medical official: 'Oh well, what can you expect when you've got MS?' Perhaps the doctor assumes you already know, so is simply being matter of fact rather than callous. Nevertheless, the shock you experience can be profound, and the effect of those words simply devastating. If this has been your experience, you know how destructive it can be. However busy medical professionals are, meticulous care must be taken to avoid this way of giving a diagnosis. Even if it was a genuine mistake, it ranks as a blunder, and the patient has every right to feel upset.

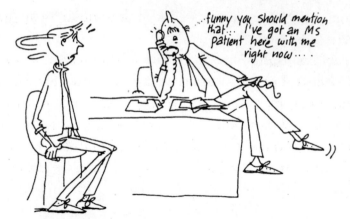

...THERE IS DOUBLE PAIN WHEN THE DIAGNOSIS IS GIVEN BADLY
IN AN OFF-HAND DISMISSIVE WAY...

What is worse, the doctor's assumption may deny you the opportunity to discuss the implications of your diagnosis because you are probably too shocked to say much. Learning that you have MS is the natural time to talk about the disease and how you are likely to be affected, so it is important that this occasion does not pass without useful comment on either side.

Fortunately, it rarely happens nowadays that a diagnosis is shared first with a partner or parent(s). That information rightfully belongs to the person with MS and should not be treated as a secret burden among relatives. When the secret is eventually revealed, perhaps years later, relationships can take such a knocking that trust is lost for ever. People with MS inevitably feel resentment if information about their health is withheld, so carers are advised to be open and honest.

Very few people with MS wish they had never been told and kept shielded from the truth. Those who do probably have a history of being unable or unwilling to cope with anything unpleasant in life. The problem lies not within the diagnosis of MS, but within their own personality.

Occasionally you hear of people who discovered their diagnosis by devious means, such as steaming open a letter or sneakily reading their medical notes. If so, they clearly needed to know and were ready to be told. It may be that some old-fashioned doctors sense this and test out their patients' readiness by allowing notes to be easily available.

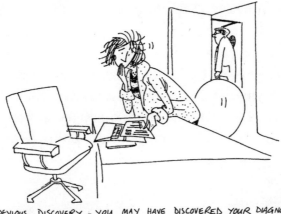

DEVIOUS DISCOVERY - YOU MAY HAVE DISCOVERED YOUR DIAGNOSIS
BY READING YOUR MEDICAL NOTES UPSIDE DOWN WHILE THE
DOCTOR WAS OUT...

If you have a certain, or even probable, diagnosis, you have the right to be told how certain or uncertain it is. Keeping back such information leads to much anger and resentment. It is a fundamentally patronizing attitude that destroys a good patient–doctor relationship. Of course, discovering your diagnosis by devious means gives you, rather than the doctor, the upper hand. You must decide whether to confront the doctor, or play dumb and wait for the revelation.

Not being told a diagnosis directly can lead to more

anxiety than is necessary. Frank, whose health care was covered by an employment scheme, was suddenly and unexpectedly refused long-term insurance, and found his cover limited to one year. A highly intelligent man with many years of first-aid experience, he assumed he must be suffering something far worse than MS. For several years he lived in a fearful twilight world, expecting each year to be his last. Frank admitted he should have asked outright, but had expected his doctor to know him well enough to tell him directly. The diagnosis of MS, when finally confirmed, gave him hope again and the promise of a much better future. He knew it was a disease that wouldn't kill him, unlike those he'd been imagining, provided he lived a balanced life with sufficient rest and relaxation to balance his demanding professional work. This has in fact been his experience. His life became full and happy because having MS was something he believed he could cope with.

When a clear diagnosis cannot yet be made

With the advent of sensitive MRI scanners that can show up multiple areas of damage, the time it takes to diagnose MS has been greatly reduced, even if you have had only one episode of symptoms. However, in non-typical cases MS may be suspected for months or years before there is sufficient objective information to make a clear and unequivocal diagnosis. This puts an almost intolerable strain on patients and their families, and a distance between them and their doctors. It may seem to you as if the doctor is holding out on you, especially if you are experiencing inexplicable symptoms.

There is a very real dilemma for any doctor who suspects MS but does not find the right combination of clinical information and test results present. A patient wants to know why his or her body isn't functioning properly, as does the doctor, who needs to rule out diseases or conditions that may be more serious or treatable.

One common occurrence among people with neurological symptoms is that they tend to become introspective. Their symptoms are frightening, and even small ones take on a great significance. As MS symptoms come and go, and are bizarre in character, those who have them can seem simply neurotic or hysterical. It follows that a doctor with such a patient may fear an increased hysterical reaction if he gives too early a diagnosis of MS, which can't be cured or systematically controlled. More often than not, though, such a patient copes quite adequately with a definite diagnosis. It is far preferable to not knowing the cause of symptoms. Left in the dark, you might imagine that valuable time is being lost – time that should be spent on treating your disorder. On diagnosis, the anxiety usually ceases to be hysterical, and assumes a natural level.

When a doctor cannot make a definite MS diagnosis with professional confidence, he should give support by assuring a patient that he has heard and accepted all the evidence given. Sometimes you have to ask your doctor to do just that. It is vital that you know you are believed and can come back again and again to discuss the matter. If your doctor can honestly admit his reason for being unable (but not unwilling) to diagnose, your relationship is one to be trusted and highly valued.

Following an MS diagnosis

What you decide to do when newly diagnosed with MS will depend on your personality and how much of a trauma the diagnosis is. You might need time and solitude to absorb and react to the diagnosis in private or with a chosen few. You might feel the need to keep it quiet for a while. You might even be determined not to reveal it to anyone at all. Perhaps you fear dismissal from work, being walked out on by your partner, being seen as a failure, or even in some way responsible for your body malfunctioning.

On the other hand, you might want to 'broadcast' the news so that other people will know immediately what is wrong. Perhaps you need others to understand what you have had to put up with and what you fear lies ahead. Maybe you need the truth out in the open because it is just too much to hold on to alone.

Between the two extremes there is a workable balance. Sharing the diagnosis invites support and caring. It gives a legitimate reason for making changes in lifestyle and redirecting energy and resources most efficiently. You are responsible for your own life, and can choose how you will relate to those in your world. You can do this well when you know how to cope with the inevitable consequences of an MS diagnosis.

Putting the past into perspective

Diagnosis is a point in life when you can dare to admit the full, uncomfortable reality of what is now an officially confirmed part of yourself. The experience of the past begins to make sense now in the light of this new information. It is a time to begin unravelling the mysteries of annoying symptoms. It can be liberating to be able to name MS as the cause of a multitude of previously isolated and unrelated incidents. A diagnosis can have the effect of clearing confusion and lifting burdens that have made life puzzling and difficult, and have soured relationships as a consequence.

A firm diagnosis justifies your behaviour: the experience prior to diagnosis was real, not simply imagined. It also buys you a breathing space; time is needed to absorb the fact that MS is part of your life ahead. In a sense, it moved in permanently long ago, and its demand for accommodation is being heard loud and clear only now.

For most people there follows a time of facing up to the facts and the challenge of starting again. The reality of MS is that you may not have enough energy to cope simultaneously with physical symptoms and the essential process of re-evaluation. However, it is helpful to tie up loose ends from the past as soon as you feel able to so that you are free to focus attention on what you need to cope with here and now. This will involve looking at many aspects of life that you have previously pushed into a corner and ignored. There is always a danger that those closest will not want stones from the past to be turned over. They may not see any necessity for change, and will cling to the status quo – or, alternatively, make a quick exit.

In a sense, every MS diagnosis is a shock. Even if it has been suspected for a long time and comes as a relief after a period of uncertainty, it is still a shock. It is a shock that numbs and feels unreal. It is a shock that enrages and seems unfair. It is a shock that can hurl you into panic and despair. It is also inescapable, and one way of dealing with such shock is to attempt to ignore its repercussions.

The discovery of new, strong and powerful feelings is as painful and confusing as discovering you have MS. Feelings make themselves obvious sooner or later. They exist, like toes or fingers, as a natural part of you. At diagnosis, you and those close to you may not know quite what you are feeling. Your feelings may seem to be out of control or getting in the way of your thinking. You may not be sure why you are reacting so strongly, nor clear what the reaction is about. Your body cannot escape the reality of feelings and their effect on it. Unhappiness or pleasure, depression or exhilaration have a consequent reaction in the body, an 'emotional tone' that cannot be ignored. Add this additional overlay to MS symptoms and diagnosis, and it's understandable that there is a confused welter of feelings and a struggle over who you are as a person right now.

In this situation the focus needs to be on finding your identity afresh. At diagnosis you take a knocking. It is almost as if you step out of your skin without a new one to step into. The only way of coping is to focus on the reality of what you feel, the way you are behaving and what symptoms you are experiencing.

It is a fact much overlooked that everyone grows up expecting to live a full life with a normal healthy body. We all seem programmed to expect stability. That is why so many elderly people are distressed by the inevitable problems of getting old. When you are young you can accept that the slowing down and gradual deterioration of the human body is a normal or natural process because it is still far off. As you become older, this change no longer seems quite as acceptable, and can be a source of anger and crisis. Similarly, when you have MS you feel affronted by its intrusive impact yet other people will readily accept your symptoms and disability as an inevitable consequence of having the disease.

So what feelings do people experience when it seems that their right to normal health has been denied and they are forced to accept a diagnosis of MS? It is perfectly normal to feel sorrow and loss, anger and frustration, fear and isolation. It is also normal to move from total denial to resignation and acceptance. Each of these feelings needs to be understood, worked through and adjusted to if you are to function smoothly again.

Feelings of sadness and loss

No loss in life can be ignored. The natural reaction to loss is to express your sorrow. Call it mourning or grieving, it is part of bereavement. Although there are some things in life people are glad to lose, it is natural to struggle, kick and fight when something valued is torn from you.

What is it you perceive you have lost when newly diagnosed with MS? It may be any or all of the following.

- You lose a normally active body and gain a body suffering from a named disease, MS.
- You lose a body that you have always believed functioned at your command, and gained a body that clearly functions in its own sweet way.

- You lose a body that is averagely active and on the go, and acquire a body that is fatigued.
- You may lose – at least temporarily – legs that hop, skip and jump, swapping them for ones that drag, limp and stumble.
- You may lose hands and arms that put on make-up or work a lathe, eyes that locate the oncoming traffic without having to turn your head, speech that is lucid and flowing, a brain that remembers in a flash and deals efficiently with impressions and situations.
- You may lose a lifestyle in which you are always in control, doing what you want, when you want, without restrictions imposed by your body.

Each of these losses may result in other losses, including self-confidence, social life, family and friends, even loss of work. When feelings of sadness in response to loss sweep over you your appetite may go, your sleep may be disturbed, you may feel depressed and despondent. What you need is to find a way of putting your life together again.

There are three steps to deal with sadness:
- Accept your sadness as a normal and healthy reaction to the loss or losses you perceive after diagnosis.
- Find ways of expressing the sadness so that it comes out into the open. Holding in sad feelings is an immense effort, and consumes the energy you need to fight MS.
- If you can trust someone to be with you when you need to talk about your losses and sorrow, it will help you to release the feelings in the most healing way.

Some people find psychotherapy helpful, and the touch of an understanding person reassuring and healing.

Dealing with loss

Loss of health is never easy to come to terms with, and cannot be ignored. If you want to go on living meaningfully, you have to adjust to it. After an MS diagnosis people will become aware of changes both physical and emotional, and in the way they relate to other people. Some of these changes will feel like losses.

It is possible to move through this time of loss and learn to adjust. It's rather like a bereavement, and involves going through various stages that take you from confusion about MS to integration of it in your life.

DENIAL

The initial reaction to loss is to deny it and refuse to believe it. You might not want to hear about MS or meet anyone else with the disease. You do all you can to prove to yourself and the world at large that you could not possibly have MS.

RESISTANCE

Then comes the resistant period, when you may be very energetic, avidly seeking advice and investigating possible cures and treatments. Inside, you admit that your MS is real, but find it hard to accept its impact. You need to find ways of beating the disease. Your energy may come across in a belligerent way, and other people may find you angry. Doctors often bear the brunt of angry outbursts, for this is the stage when those newly diagnosed feel they have a right to know about their illness, particularly any details of how it is likely to progress, and their doctors may not be giving them, or may not have, all the answers.

ADJUSTMENT

Once the reality of an MS diagnosis is faced, however reluctantly, a person begins to feel in control of life again, learning how to cope with feelings, even if they are negative ones, and recognizing what it is like to feel isolated emotionally too. It is a bargaining stage in which the aim is to win the battle between accepting that what is left is actually good and letting go of what has gone. It takes determination to emphasize the positive, but it is a good way of overcoming depression. When you are willing to disclose that you have MS and what that means for you, you help others to respond more appropriately. It helps to reach out for support from others, whether they be individuals or groups that focus on coming to terms with MS. The sooner you accept whatever practical support and help you want, and thus start adjusting to having MS, the better your quality of life will be. What must be remembered with MS, however, is that this affirming process is often interrupted by relapses. Just as you feel you are able to cope, you suffer a setback, and may find yourself back at the denial or resistance stage. It is rather like a game of snakes and ladders.

ACCEPTANCE

The final stage of the bereavement process is when a person is able to accept MS and all it entails simply as part of life. By now it is possible to negotiate some of the needs a person with MS has in order to fit in with the requirements of others. MS is no longer the total preoccupation, but can be integrated into everyday life alongside other people. It is no longer something to be ashamed of, and people find they can ask for and receive the help and support they need.

Going through the process of bereavement is one that family and friends need to experience as much as the person with MS. What is special about adjusting to the disease is that you may have to do it more than once. All is well until the next relapse or bad patch comes along, then the process begins all over again. Despite that, if you have once adjusted well to MS, you will be able to do so again, working through the stages, even if they are slow and painful, because you already know the relief that comes at the end.

What happens if you *don't* mourn your loss(es) in some way, or get stuck at one of the stages, is that your life may well become less rich and satisfying. On top of having MS, you may also feel depressed. You may lose sleep and appetite. Feelings of despondency may increase, and lead to your feeling less than positive about yourself. If this pattern continues, you'll start to see yourself in a different – and negative – light, and will be likely to push to one side formerly valued plans and goals for the future. There will probably be a negative effect on your relationships too, for with depression come feelings of rejection by others and an increasing sense of isolation. Instead of growing to maturity, your personality will tend to stagnate and you will find yourself taking on the stereotyped behaviour of a depressed person who believes that MS is the end of the road.

Only by facing up to the losses that are an inevitable part of your MS and mourning them properly can you avoid a downward spiral into depression and be able to move upwards instead.

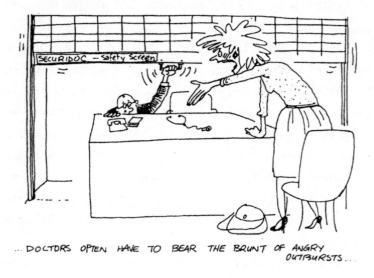

... DOCTORS OFTEN HAVE TO BEAR THE BRUNT OF ANGRY OUTBURSTS ...

Feelings of anger and frustration

Anger is a natural reaction when something you want to do is not possible. MS may stop many of your goals from being realized, and blocked goals result in frustration. This holds true whether you or your partner has the disease.

What do you do with this anger? Where should it be directed? How should it be released? The two natural reactions to anger are either to fight back or run away.

Not acknowledging you are angry and holding on to it is unnatural and unhelpful. It may be better to:

- Accept anger as a normal and healthy reaction.
- Own your anger, and take responsibility for handling it in such a way that it does not harm you or anyone else. It can become a source of creative energy.
- Find safe and, if possible, productive ways of expressing these strong feelings. You may need to seek professional help from someone trained in psychotherapy to get started. If you have the physical energy, you might find that a vigorous activity, such as polishing the car, digging the garden or kneading dough, is an excellent release of anger and frustration. If you are low in energy, you will not believe that you can gain any benefit from using up that last ounce of 'go' on bothering to express your frustration. However, if you have the courage or are desperate enough to try, you will find that a roar of frustration or a defiant shake of the fist will result in a physiological release of tension that is followed by a doubled resurgence of energy.
- Don't throw your anger at someone else and try to get him or her to take the blame. Again, own your feelings of anger, and your right to feel that way when what you want is denied. MS adds to life's frustrations, but doesn't give you the right to lash out at family, friends and doctors when you feel angry.
- If there is something you can do to change and improve the situation, work first of all on dealing healthily with the angry feelings. When they are released you will have energy and a clearer mind to think of what options are open and the best way of going round the blocked goal.

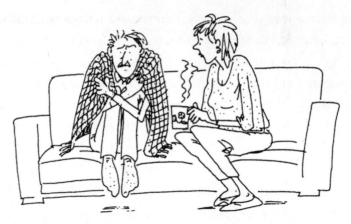

CURLING UP SMALL, A BLANKET WRAPPED ROUND TIGHTLY, AND WITH SOMEONE CARING THERE AS SUPPORT, WORKS WELL

The effect of fear

Fear can have a paralysing effect, or wildly accelerate you into panic. An MS diagnosis is a fearful one because the disease has fluctuating symptoms and a variable course: no one can be certain what will happen. It is normal to be fearful in the face of the unknown. A faith or deeply held philosophy of life, and the support of loving people, can help contain the fear. So too can allowing yourself to be brave enough to look at the threat you are facing.

Talking through what would be the worst that could happen, and asking yourself what you would do then, very often results in the unexpected discovery that although unwelcome, the threat can be coped with. It won't remove the threat, but it will make it clear, and will release energy to cope with finding alternatives, if they exist. Better a single devil you've tracked to its lair than a score of imaginary goblins in every dark corner.

Sometimes you can't voice what your fear is, or can't

pin it down. If you have someone close who wants to be supportive, you might like to try asking for physical reassurance by being held close. Curling up small and being wrapped tightly in a blanket, while someone caring sits alongside for support, works well. It is a natural, child-like action that the body responds to in its own time by slowly relaxing.

MS diagnosis and crisis

At diagnosis you find yourself faced with new information about yourself. It forces you to take stock, consider new challenges and discover strategies to help you cope.

You could say it is a time of crisis. For a time after diagnosis, you and those close to you are caught up in a unique situation. Temporarily, you may feel as if you are encapsulated in a bubble, isolated, cut off from the mainstream, halted, until you have had sufficient opportunity to reassess where you are, who you are and what direction you wish to go in. Every MS diagnosis produces shock waves that flood into every aspect of your life, and ripple on to affect the lives of others you come into contact with, however fleetingly. Until the ripples have calmed down, the crisis continues.

What you experience at diagnosis may be your only crisis time with MS – or you might find that other crises follow. Much depends on the sort of person you are and the way you normally deal with unexpected situations. And, of course, it also depends on how your MS develops. It makes a world of difference if you are able to face the crisis and discover ways of coping with MS that work for you. If you leave the crisis of diagnosis unresolved, it could mark the start of a long stage of conflict inside yourself.

What exactly is a crisis situation like? How do you know if you are going through a crisis? You first experience some signs of stress, and these can be physical or psychological or both. You tend to react in one of two ways: either you panic, or you feel like throwing in the towel. You feel overwhelmed, somewhat helpless and inadequate. It's not surprising, then, that you can't tackle life with your usual enthusiasm and efficiency. All you want is to get rid of the uncomfortable feeling of being knocked off balance, which is what crisis is about. It's too painful an experience for you to want to prolong it, so there is a temptation to run from it and hide.

The other side of a positive diagnosis is the relief it brings. On the one hand, it is so unexpected and devastating; but on the other, you now know that you were right in your suspicions. One moment it feels like the worst day of your life, the next you feel it's better to know. For a while it seems like your whole world is tumbling in; then suddenly you recognize 'better the devil you know'. Initially you may feel there's no point in going on; but once you've taken the diagnosis on board, you begin to feel that you can now get on and live again. Instead of wanting to run away, you begin to accept that it's time to change and rebuild.

However you react, you register that having MS spells change. Nothing will be quite the same again. You will still be all you were before, positive and negative, but you will have a new and different perspective. This is the crux of the crisis around diagnosis. Even if it is a relief to have a name for your health problem, you still go through a time of crisis as you are forced to take stock.

Even if your MS is currently benign, you will still need to consider a fresh perspective on life. This could mean changing your priorities, accepting less ambitious goals, or at least being prepared to achieve them in a different way and with less pressure on time and energy. Until you have made a reassessment of this sort, you are still in crisis.

Sometimes a diagnosis is revealed at a time when you are experiencing a considerable number of symptoms, a run of relapses, or increasing disability. Some symptoms have a direct effect on whether you can drive, work, socialize or continue to care for yourself independently. This is obviously a major crisis situation too.

It is also a time of crisis for family and friends. They want to support you, and at the same time they have their own reactions and feelings to cope with. They experience the same range of emotions as the person with MS: anger about the unfairness and inconvenience of MS; sorrow over the pain and lost opportunities; fear of the unknown. On top of this, there is often guilt because they don't have the disease and you do. Their relationship with you – and yours with them – will be affected as you each work through the crisis. They might try to 'make it better', or they might 'want out' at once. You need both time and a strategy to cope with the crisis. This subject is dealt with in more detail in Chapter 4.

THREE

Learning to live with MS

When forced to deal with a difficult situation, people talk about 'coping', as if that in itself is a ready-made solution. Of course it isn't, but it does help you to find ways of living with the problem and minimizing its effects. Coping strategies are very much an individual matter, and can be broadly divided into two categories: change and management.

The first of these – change – is a very good way of coping because it alters the situation to suit your needs. Sometimes this can remove the problem completely. Unfortunately, this is not true of MS. Despite its very changeable nature – in the sense that it comes and goes – MS is not going to go away. You cannot choose not to have it around any longer.

As far as MS is concerned, the only changes you can make are not to the disease itself but your reactions to it. The situation doesn't change – your thoughts and feelings about it do. This is the management approach to coping. You may be unable to change the way your body behaves with MS, but you can learn to manage the way you react to it. This will not be a new skill to you, for all your life you have been managing your reactions to a host of situations. In this sense, MS is just another new challenge for you to face, and you bring to it your previous coping skills – sharpened for most effective use.

Strategies for coping

There are basically three ways of coping with MS. The first is to plan ahead right now, while you have the energy to build up the resources you will need for what lies ahead. This is a management strategy in which you anticipate the future, making plans for a rainy day. Given the fact of your MS, what are you likely to need in the future to help you cope as well as possible? Only you know what resources you would like to develop within yourself. The nature of MS means that it really helps to learn how to be at peace with the person you are. Some people find this possible through relaxation classes, meditation or a religious faith.

When you have MS it also helps to find ways of maintaining your dignity as a person who knows what you want and is able to ask for it straight. It is therefore important to learn how to make decisions well, and to feel at ease in your relationships with other people. Whatever enables you to be in control of who you are and how well you relate to others can improve your quality of life.

There is also some practical forward planning you might wish to consider. For example, if you are thinking of moving house, it might be wise to choose one that offers easy access for a wheelchair, or that has a downstairs cloakroom. Forward planning is an immensely practical skill in the process of coping.

The second coping strategy is to learn how to cushion yourself against the realities of MS. You can do this by denying or ignoring what is happening because to face up to it is more than you can handle at that time. Alternatively, you can count your blessings. This can be hard if MS is affecting you badly, but it can help if you are prepared to admit openly that there are people who are worse off. It is inevitable with a disease like MS that there will be dark times physically and psychologically, when, as it were, you need to go into neutral and coast along for a while. This isn't a time to sort things out, but to be cosseted and snuggled with cushions while the bleakness passes. You can pick up whatever concerns you at a later time, when you feel strong enough to deal with it again.

The third coping strategy is to face up to what is actually happening to you right here and now. This demands that you take responsibility for the way you react, feel and think, and it works by helping you to reach out for support from those who care about you.

You will need to use each of these coping strategies at different times. What matters is not so much whether your attempts to cope are successful or not, but that you try. This has its own positive spin-off.

Overcoming helplessness

There will be times when you feel helpless – perhaps because you are physically dependent on others to care for you, or need much more practical help than previously to cope with daily life. On the other hand, you might feel helpless because you have reached a low ebb emotionally and feel drained of all resources. Living with fatigue and other MS symptoms can be wearisome, and it is natural to respond by wondering whether or not you have the resources to pull through. At times like these you are likely to feel helpless, but that feeling will eventually pass. It is important not to panic when you feel helpless, but to accept it as a temporary imbalance.

Falling into the trap of paying too much attention to these feelings of helplessness is easy, but can be damaging. If you indulge yourself in always anticipating the worst and feed off the helplessness those thoughts engender, you will soon find yourself stuck in a negative way of thinking. This will discolour the whole of your life. It will make you prone to repeated spells of mild depression, and you may even find yourself wanting to chuck it all in and accept a submissive exit from life. This was Dorothy's experience. She believed she had lost a psychological battle with herself, and as a result felt out of control of her own life. Her deep sense of helplessness made her think her MS symptoms were worse than they really were. In her helplessness, she behaved in character with her feelings; she neglected her health, didn't eat properly and found she wasn't sleeping well. She isolated herself from the support of family, friends and doctor.

Research with cancer patients has shown that feelings of helplessness and end-of-the-road pessimism may actually hamper the immune system. This factor is also likely to be significant in MS. It is not feeling helpless for a while that matters. It is remaining helpless and no longer believing you can do anything to change it that really knocks you back.

Dealing with stress

Stress is one of those inevitable concomitants of modern life, and much talked about in negative terms. However, stress isn't only negative. It comes in a variety of guises, and in a positive light can act as a challenge that forces you to change or make adjustments. While stress can give purpose to what you do, it can also be too much of a good thing. It becomes negative when you dig in your heels and fail to make the adjustments required. Confront stress with refusal to act and there's a difficult time ahead. It is not really stress that is the problem, but the way you handle it. The key is your ability to adjust to or cope with stress.

Events that have a stressful effect include many everyday experiences, such as moving house, getting married and having a baby, all of which are associated with pleasure and fun too. Exams, tensions at work and taking on new responsibilities are stresses accepted by

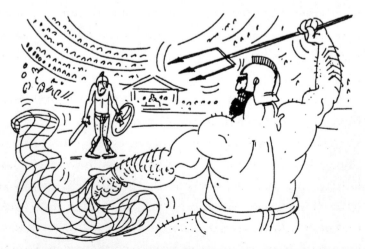

...CONFRONT STRESS WITH A REFUSAL TO ACT AND THERE'S A DIFFICULT TIME AHEAD !

many as part of a lifestyle choice. Unanticipated worries, such as conflict within close relationships, divorce, unemployment, accidents, severe illness and death, bring stress everyone would rather avoid. Each stressful event has a physical, emotional and/or social effect.

There is no doubt that the way you perceive stress has a direct effect on your health. The extent of its effect depends on how long the stress lasts, how intensely it is experienced, and, most significantly, on how susceptible as an individual you are to it. This, in turn, is determined by your personality and the support you need. Stressful situations can provoke you to anger so that you fight back, or arouse fear that makes you want to run away and hide. The most dangerous reactions to stress are feelings of hopelessness and helplessness. When you feel unable to cope for a period of time, your body is more likely to have abnormal or lowered immune responses. This can precipitate the appearance of symptoms and the onset of disease. Many body mechanisms react negatively to a helpless reaction to stress. It makes good sense, then, once you have MS, to check that you are giving yourself the best chance, and to learn how to cope well.

Evidence is occasionally quoted that some people with MS have experienced three times the average number of stressful life events in a two-year period prior to early MS symptoms appearing. Poor handling of these stresses, it is suggested, perhaps helps trigger the disease. Once you have MS, the way you deal with even temporary stress may precipitate exacerbations, so you need to take stock and check that you are developing skilful ways of coping with it.

Accepting help

Most people enjoy their independence not merely for the sense of freedom it brings, but also because they need to feel in control. When control is threatened, we do all we can to get it back, as if unsure of who we are if taken out of the driving seat. Reluctance to accept help and care is normal, especially among people with chronic conditions. We hate feeling beholden to others, and find it easier to give help than receive it ourselves. However, we are usually glad of help that meets a specific need at just the right time. Fortunately, people are generally brilliant at responding to a crisis, but only if they know about it.

Nonetheless, getting help at the right time can be a problem because MS is so unpredictable, with stamina varying from day to day, or even hour to hour. Whenever we run out of energy, struggle with coordination and motor skills, and experience emotional and cognitive lows, we really could do with a hand at that point. When at low ebb, we may be less than tactful, and our request for help can come across as a demand. So if our MS lands us with a string of crises that merge into an ongoing need for more regular support, it makes sense to plan such help and care wisely. It's about learning new skills. Although professional carers are taught how to care, few of us with MS are informed about what types of care and support are available and appropriate in different circumstances, or, more significantly, how to negotiate receiving it. Care is best arranged on mutually agreeable terms, which means that both the carer and the cared for must have an equal say in the negotiation. Inevitably, individual preferences are important, but it's often a matter of trying things out in order to discover what works best. Many people conserve energy by seeking help early on rather than wearing themselves out trying to achieve an impossible task. They can then use the reserved energy more profitably and pleasurably in other activities. For example, vacuuming the house may be delegated to someone else while you read a bedtime story to your children. This approach to help is about maintaining a presence that reflects who we really are deep down.

A common fear around accepting help is feeling placed at a disadvantage. It's not a question of being ungrateful: it's more to do with our personal difficulty in acknowledging that we are visibly different and needy, and not wanting to depend on others. It is never easy to admit we can no longer do certain things for ourselves. You may even suspect that some will be glad of an opportunity to demonstrate how caring they are. Nobody wants to receive pity. It takes self-confidence to believe that accepting help appropriately is positive and does not reflect on who you really are. Your value as an individual lies outside such matters. However, you can enhance relationships by learning how best to ask for help, stating what you want directly and pleasantly. You cannot expect anyone to mind-read. By treating others with honesty and respect, you will make it possible for them to treat you similarly.

Coping with your partner

MS is a demanding disease, so it is not unusual for it to have a negative effect on relationships. Sadly, there is plenty of evidence that divorce and separation are high among couples where one partner has MS. Any crisis, illness or otherwise, will inevitably hit the most vulnerable spot, and this is most dramatically true in close relationships. In theory, the one person you can hope to be closest to, best understood by, cared for and loved by is your partner – and this may be your experience. But it could be that your relationship has never reached such intimacy, and never will. You may be enjoying a secure, fulfilling relationship, or putting up with one already cracking with stress and strain. MS is going to force the issue, if .there is one.

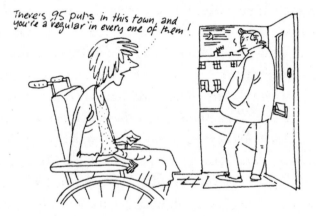

MS WILL INEVITABLY HIT THE MOST VULNERABLE SPOT
IN A RELATIONSHIP...

However, it is too easy to blame MS for souring a relationship. The disease itself is not to blame, but it can be a trigger. It puts your partnership under a harsh spotlight that picks out its existing weaknesses as well as its strengths. What counts is how well you and your partner got on before the diagnosis. If you skated along without ever needing to resolve any major issues, MS is one that really tests your mettle. If all you have ever done is to confront problem after problem, MS can become just one more to work on, or one too many. The disease can become the focus of a struggle you are already waging in which, once again, you try to resolve the inequalities in your relationship. Some use it to force a change in the other so that their way of maintaining the relationship can win. This time the stakes are high, and there is the potential for far-reaching damage to be done to both partners. This is a good time to evaluate realistically what your relationship consists of, and to assess what each of you is willing to contribute to its success.

Both you and your partner must come to terms with the extent to which you are able to cope with MS. Your experience of it will be shared, but from a different perspective. You will both struggle with strong feelings – feelings that may be kept firmly under control, but equally may seep out or explode. You may find yourself wanting to lash out at your partner or keep a distance, to protect or reject, and often to manipulate. It takes courage to admit that with MS you both hurt. That is the way it was for Janet, who looked after her husband with devoted care and took over the role of breadwinner when, in his later years, he became severely disabled. David could never talk to her or anyone else about his MS. They coped, accepting the strain of never daring to say aloud what a hell of a disease MS had become. After David's death Janet needed to share her hatred of what living with MS was like. She made particular mention of how normal he had looked from the waist up but how much notice she had taken of his hands, which in his late sixties had become visibly twisted. She hated the memory of those hands; for her they symbolized the disability of MS. Physical disability and day-to-day nursing care get to partners. They suffer. They agonize when they give all they can, knowing it will never repair the disability. It is pointless trying to decide who gets the worst deal. Both of you do.

It is an indisputable fact that while you cannot escape your MS, your partner may want to – and decide to. Only a small minority walk out early on, without giving you and your MS a go. But we all differ in what we are prepared to put up with. It can happen that sickness and disability are the very things your partner most fears and really cannot cope with. Anything else would be all right, but not something like MS. Some have already been looking for an excuse to leave, and in MS find one they can justify. However, it can work the other way round too. Maria quickly made up her mind upon her diagnosis that although she was prepared to cope with having MS, she was not prepared to put up with her husband too. She immediately started divorce proceedings. Sometimes the opposite happens, and a partner stays in a troubled relationship because to leave it would mean coping with too much guilt.

There are certain factors that help to cement a relationship and give it a sound enough basis for both partners to incorporate MS.

Agree . . . as far as you are able, that you are going to work together to come to terms with MS. Neither of you can afford to deny its existence and its impact on your relationship; no relationship works well if reality is ignored.

Improve . . . communication with each other. While it will also be important to communicate with other people and gain their support, the most important relationship is the one with your partner. Communicating well is tough, and there is always room for improvement. It is worth seeking advice and learning new skills. There are books to consult, professionals to talk to and courses available on how to improve the way you relate to others. Good communication is the best antidote to an ailing relationship. Once you start working together on that, you will find yourselves able to deal with difficulties frankly, handle conflict constructively, and to seek new options when the old ways are no longer practicable.

Dare . . . to be the person you are, to accept that you have the right to be different, that you are allowed to feel what you feel, to take the space you need to thrive in and to ask for your needs to be met. Because you need acceptance and fear rejection, you can easily slip into the position of covering up your needs and inadequacies. To be honest and open about them may sound a tall order, but it is a worthwhile goal. It puts the responsibility on you first to know yourself, and then to invite your partner to respond. It is important to emphasize that your partner always has the right to say that he or she can meet some, a few or none of your needs at any given time. You have the same right. The value of expressing your needs and feelings is not to demand that they be fulfilled, but to communicate them honestly in an unthreatening way. If you both know what is going on, you can make an honest response and face up to the consequences without having to spend time imagining what the other is thinking and feeling. Trying to mind-read is impossible anyway, and eats up anxious hours.

One of the things that upsets good communication in a relationship is not being able to express your true feelings. This is not easy for most people at the best of times, and when MS is part of the scene it is particularly difficult. Feelings and fears of dependency cause extra strains in the relationship, which can result in feelings of anger, fear and sadness. If these emotions are bottled up rather than expressed, you may find a distance developing between you and your partner. Deprived of closeness, you may feel rejected, may deny or overprotect, may manipulate and feel guilty. Sometimes this can escalate to a point where your relationship is damaged or destroyed.

Alternatively, one or both of you may find the strain so great that you want to take it out on the other – or yourself – and may behave in an anti-social, self-destructive way, such as taking to drink. A few will contemplate suicide. If any of these reactions become part of your relationship, you need to take stock of what is happening and get help to resolve them. Counselling may prove helpful in facing your feelings and working them through.

The most explosive feeling is anger, a very common emotion in MS relationships, but one rarely admitted to. Anger is a natural reaction when you are frustrated in your attempts to achieve a goal. You may bottle up your frustrations until you become tense and unable to share them easily. You are crowded in by them, and experience unpleasant negative reactions to others, especially your partner. You can find yourself exploding with frustration when you feel you should be able to achieve something very simple and can't, and similar feelings may be experienced if your partner suggests, even mildly, that you should do something you sense you cannot. It is frustrating not to be able to do what you used to do so easily. It takes time to adjust to limitations, just as it does to find new ways around the blocks. It is only by venting the frustration without violence that you can release the energy of the anger and focus on other options and activities.

It is noticeable how often tense, angry feelings are experienced before an MS exacerbation. You may not be conscious of physical feelings of ill-ease, and may interpret them in a psychological way because your irritability interferes with your relationship. It is almost as if you are searching for a psychological explanation of vague physical sensations still in the background, unable yet to pinpoint and label the existence of hidden symptoms until they emerge fully. In the meantime, your body is already reacting and under tension. It takes very little then to trigger an outburst of angry feelings. (People react in a similar way when they are coming down with a cold.) It therefore helps if you and your partner can keep alert to this hidden cause of anger or irritability. Since it is, in the main, physiologically based, it does not warrant being made into an issue between you.

There is a good side to anger, and that is when you can channel the frustrations you feel about MS into constructive and creative outlets. Anger does not have to be expressed in damaging ways: it can instead push you and your partner into doing something worthwhile. It's the good anger that energizes you to take part in a backgammon marathon, do a parachute jump, organize a charity fashion show or sit in your wheelchair and collect funds for MS research and welfare.

If you live with a chronic illness, it is likely to have some effect on your personality because you put up with it day in and day out. If your chronic illness is a neurological one like MS, the neurological damage may result in a further impact on your personality. Demyelination in MS can interfere with your emotions, your mental faculties, your memory and your concentration. The lesions causing this may have a permanent effect, or simply produce temporary fluctuations, so the impact on your personality may either be very subtle, or so pronounced that it could be taken for bloody-mindedness. You may not realize there is any change in you, but, in much the same way that a teetotaller observes the effects of alcohol on a drinker, your partner may notice it. He or she needs to understand that your MS can exaggerate what you are feeling. You may feel low and depressed or unusually bright and cheerful in the face of adversity. Your MS may affect your ability to think straight and reason soundly. You may feel out of balance with yourself, as if you are only partially in control. It's a lot for one body to cope with, and if, as a result, you become more introspective or self-centred than usual, your partner may misread this as selfishness. You may not realize that at such times you become abrasive, critical and insensitive to the point of hurting others and yourself, but your partner will. He or she may want to confront you about negative changes in your attitude, and try to make you change back again. If the change is due to MS, there is a limit to how much you can do until the inflammation causing the exacerbation passes. It is wisest not to make too much of it. It becomes a more worrying problem if MS has a permanent and negative effect on your personality. In this case, it is important for the partner to blame the MS, not the person, who needs special understanding and love.

As MS symptoms often limit what you can and cannot do, you may find yourself forced into new roles in a relationship. This may have a disruptive effect. It is humiliating no longer to be able to do what you have previously counted important and pleasurable. It is also frustrating for your partner not to be able to rely on you for certain things. Not being able to work, to get about independently or to maintain a satisfying sexual relationship in the way you used to are bound to result in feelings of tension and guilt until both of you have had time to adjust. But being forced to change the nature of your role in a relationship is not an insurmountable barrier, and need not be used as an excuse to break up. It is good to give yourself and your partner space to try on 'new hats', experimenting to see how best the two of you can cope together. Your partner might be keen to help you strike a balance between what you can manage to do and how realistic it is to exert that amount of energy on achieving it. This can become quite a crucial issue during exacerbations, relapses and longer spells of disabling symptoms. It helps if you can talk over your priorities together, and assess what your energy level and physical skills are. Since the latter vary with MS, it is your priorities that need checking to see whether they are still viable.

This became an issue for Eileen while she was getting over an attack and could not face having people round. She had previously had a great reputation for serving wonderful home-made meals. Now she wasn't well enough to do any food preparation, she always found some excuse not to entertain, but felt very guilty about it. It was only after friends began dropping in unexpectedly and simple meals were rustled up with everyone's help that Eileen began to see her real priority was being able to welcome guests to the relaxed atmosphere of the home. With her husband's help, she became clear what her priority in entertaining was, and together they found alternative ways of offering hospitality. It nonetheless took her a long time to accept that she was not responsible for having MS and did not need to feel guilty.

It can be hard to accept that disability and relapses may force you to be dependent on your partner and others for physical care (washing, feeding and so on), but this need not prevent you remaining a person in your own right. If you feel you are being 'done to' rather than 'doing', it is easy to slip into becoming dependent on your partner and letting feelings of dependency grow. This upsets the equality of your relationship. On the other hand, if you fear losing your independence, you may so fight against being helped that you never let your partner do anything for you, even when it would be natural to do so. Accepting help can be an embarrassment, particularly if you are shy about your bodily functions, yet need help in getting washed, going to the toilet or dealing with a menstrual period. Every relationship is different in its balance of dependence and independence, and there is always room for you to discover what is most appropriate for you and your partner now. The most natural person to turn to is usually your partner, and after that to a professional carer, such as a nurse.

Your partner may feel uncomfortable or reluctant to provide intimate nursing on a regular basis. This does not mean your partner does not care, but rather that he or she finds nursing care difficult. In fact, there are definite long-term advantages to opting for professional support as soon as you are unable to manage your own personal care without help. It can, for example, help you and your partner to maintain a more intimate and loving relationship, as the sexual side of things can be impaired if your partner permanently becomes nurse rather than lover. What counts with MS is your ability to remain your own person and to relate to others, and it is this that will allow you and your partner to grow together in your own special way. When Tom insisted on struggling through the snow from the house to the car with a walking-frame one bitter winter, he nearly got frostbite, but gained nothing else. Using a wheelchair was quicker, warmer, lost him no dignity and gave him energy to enjoy being out with his partner.

There is a fine line between being cared for on your terms and being smothered with unwanted attention. If your partner is the sort of person who cares for you too readily when you can manage reasonably well yourself, it may be that he or she is responding to his or her own needs and not yours. He or she may be compensating for

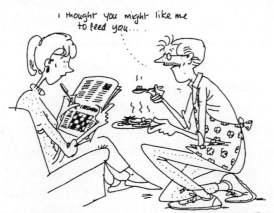

IF YOUR PARTNER IS THE SORT OF PERSON WHO CARES FOR YOU TOO READILY WHEN YOU CAN MANAGE REASONABLY WELL YOURSELF . . . .

what are perceived to be your disadvantages. You may even feel you are being hurried along into permanent disability. The end result is a relationship based on domination, in which your partner gets the upper hand, so to speak, by pushing you to accept a dependent role. If you are discouraged from doing anything much yourself, you may come to believe you no longer can, and may feel resentful. Jenni's husband was the model of a caring husband and did everything for her. His sudden death left her helpless, but in time she discovered she could manage on her own, and enjoyed being able to look after herself. Smothering has no place in a good relationship.

Occasionally, a partner chooses to ignore any information about MS in general and your MS in particular, in some cases being unpleasantly surly with it. Such a partner wants to make it clear that MS changes nothing in your relationship, and just doesn't want to know about it. Partners like this are either totally inconsiderate and selfish, or too hurt to be supportive. They cope by denying reality, and leave you feeling utterly rejected and depressed. Such extremes are rare, but far commoner are partners who sidestep involvement with MS, hoping that it will go away if you don't mention it again. They shut their ears when anyone tries to tell them about the invisible symptoms of MS, especially fatigue. They ignore any warnings you give about how much it can hurt to be touched when you are suffering from impaired sensation, or what pain you suffer from being jolted about in a wheelchair because they won't bother to learn to handle one properly. Such insensitivity and denial place intolerable stresses on a relationship. Your options are to put up with it or to get out quickly.

Partners are equally responsible for maintaining a relationship. In the new situation with MS, you can both choose to grow together in a special closeness, or struggle in a mesh of conflict. Take time to re-evaluate what you are willing to give to your partner and decide what is realistic. It is important to seek help whenever necessary, for there are times when an impartial outsider with the right skills is a better source of support for you both. Daring to explore new options can result in a most rewarding and exciting life together.

Coping with pregnancy

You and your partner have the right to choose whether or not to have a child. It has to be your joint decision. Only you know how much you really want your own children. As responsible parents, and given the unpredictable course of MS, you will assess what this might mean. Bringing up children is rewarding and fun, but it is exhausting and demanding too. You need a lot of energy and patience, and it helps to have sound finances. MS is not hereditary, but you need to appreciate that you could pass on an increased genetic susceptibility to the disease. The risk of a child born to an MS parent actually developing MS is slight – two in 100. So most children born to parents affected by MS will not inherit the condition – 980 out of 1000 are MS-free, compared with 997 out of 1000 in the general population. Few doctors would therefore consider MS in a pregnant woman or her partner as grounds for terminating a pregnancy.

Most women with MS seem to do well during pregnancy,

like most women everywhere: some bloom and others feel rough. Pregnancy won't protect you against all MS symptoms, but neither will MS prevent you experiencing a normal pregnancy. Many women report little change in the pattern of their MS during the first half of pregnancy, but find improvement in the second half, with noticeably fewer exacerbations or relapses. This is probably to do with the way the body automatically becomes mildly immuno-suppressant to protect the unborn child, which is typical of MS and other auto-immune diseases.

It is wise to plan your pregnancy. If you can conceive while in remission, or wait a couple of years after a severe relapse, you give yourself and your baby a good start. It is also important for you and your doctor to review any drugs you may be taking so that you can weigh up any possible risks. Unfortunately, little information is available about drug risks to foetuses because clinical trials are neither recommended nor considered ethical during pregnancy. Most prospective mothers err on the side of caution, as do GPs, who usually advise not taking drugs 3–6 months prior to conception, or at least opting for safer ones, if available. Staying off drugs for the first three months of pregnancy, while the unborn child's organs are developing, is also advisable.

Birth and afterwards

A mother with MS can expect to experience a normal delivery. If necessary, the midwife and doctor will be prepared to manage any weakness or spasms in the legs, and would also arrange for special help in rare cases of severe paralysis. If you need a Caesarean section, you need not worry that it will have a negative effect on the baby or your MS. *General anaesthetics* are considered safe, though many mothers with MS have C-sections with an epidural, which is also preferred for pain control.

Following the birth of your baby, you need to take extra care of yourself because there does seem to be an increased risk of relapse. It is almost as if your body has been storing up the effects of MS until after the birth. What follows is normally a period of exacerbation or relapse(s), and you are most likely to settle down to your usual pre-pregnant MS condition within a year from conception. You are less likely to experience a relapse if your MS is stable prior to conception than if it were active.

Although you may not be able to stop a relapse from happening, you can do something to make it less likely and less severe. Find out what makes you tired, what aggravates your MS symptoms, and avoid these triggers. It is vital to get as much sleep and relaxation as you possibly can – you really can't get too much. Remember that breast-feeding can be very tiring for any mother, and causes some to feel anxious. It may be worth changing to an alternative way of feeding. All women benefit from practical help and understanding support as they adjust to motherhood. You deserve as much as you can get for the sake of your health, your baby and your family. This is the time to capitalize on every labour-saving device possible.

Your priority must be yourself and your baby, for the bonding you achieve now provides the best start in life. Of course, you will sometimes feel insecure about being a mother. Most women do, and MS gives you an additional reason to feel that way. Mothers with MS often worry that the fatigue, exacerbations and relapses induced by the disease will stop them from being good mothers. In the end, your baby thrives because you are close and affectionate when you are together, even for short spells. It is the relationship that counts most; your baby really couldn't care less who does the housework, washing or cooking, so save your energy for your baby and get help with the rest.

When you feel ready, it is important for your child's development to include other loving people in his or her world. This may be an especially important safeguard for times when MS may limit your energy and full availability. Children naturally have big, loving hearts, and respond to warmth and affection from other members of the family and friends. They deserve early on to have access to additional support and security when you may not be able to do a supermum act.

No problem is too trivial to seek help for. Sometimes local mother and baby groups can be an invaluable source of reassurance and support. You need to know how much of what you are experiencing is the norm for *all* mothers; it's so easy to blame MS, and then to feel isolated and alone, an additional burden to carry. Remember, sharing what you are going through with your young baby will not only help you but support other mothers too.

Coping with children

It is sometimes said that when one member of the family becomes ill, the whole family is affected. That effect need not be negative – it can be a positive, wholesome one.

With MS you can still be the caring and considerate parent who passes on the lessons in life that matter most, as well as values and skills to last a lifetime. No parent can give more than he or she has received and experienced, and MS, for all its disadvantages, does force you to take stock and re-evaluate your life – an extra, enriching experience, the value of which can easily be overlooked.

A parent with MS often worries that his or her children will be missing out on proper care and attention, outings, the rough and tumble of games and family fun. There is some truth in this, of course, but it does not mean that their upbringing will be any less adequate than the average. Children are highly practical, and if given adequate information, they understand quickly what you can and cannot do. They have a right to know what MS means in language they understand so that they can make sense of what's going on. They often become more anxious when denied knowledge about what you are experiencing, or about any hospital visits or tests you need. Far from shielding them from MS, you are exposing them to it. Their natural sensitivity may enable them to pick up what is implied but left unsaid, or they may jump to conclusions more alarming than reality. There will be times to involve them in major family decisions so that they don't feel excluded and resentful. Sometimes they take the blame for the way you behave with MS, and suppose that they are a burden. You may be the sort who soldiers on past your fatigue level until you find yourself getting ratty and snapping at them. Your mood swings then intensify as you push yourself over the top, trying to prove you are a 'normal' parent. There are children who believe their bad behaviour may have caused you to have an attack; they may even start to feel guilty for having been born. While it may be true that your MS symptoms appeared after your child's birth, remember to give reassurance that he or she wasn't responsible for their appearance.

Children tend to go one of two ways: they either seek to separate themselves from their MS parent or both parents, or they throw themselves into helping like 'little adults'. Some are embarrassed to be seen out with a disabled parent. They may express their envy of friends whose parents don't have MS, in much the same way as some poor kids envy rich ones. This is hurtful, but a common reaction at a certain age and for certain personalities. Sometimes the fact that a parent can't do something the way other mothers and fathers can get blown out of all proportion. It is sad when a father who's loved kicking a ball about with his children can no longer do so, and yet it needn't spell disaster in their relationship. What children are often really reacting to when they seem to fuss about not having a footballer of a dad is the unspoken self-blame and disappointment of the parent. Perhaps your children are taking their cue from you. If you can admit your disappointment, accept it and move on to emphasize the positive aspects of your relationship, your child will feel he has gained from you rather than losing out. Other children are very protective, and find ways of speaking out about MS so that their friends and neighbours understand better.

While keeping children informed about your health, it is important not to treat them as mini-adults. It is one thing to encourage them to do additional household chores, but it is quite another to lean on them for emotional support and comfort. They are your children, not your peers or equals, and it is always your responsibility, as much as possible, to care for and make adequate provision for them. Children are very accommodating, and help willingly if they know they are really loved. Their respect for you must never be abused by trying to get them to side with you against others, and take on an adult role to fight for you. It is essential that you develop a network of other supports – family, friends, doctors, nurses and paramedics, social workers, clergymen, the local branch of a society concerned with MS or general disability problems (see page 284), and other people with MS. These are the proper sources of adult support, not your children.

Coping with parents

Parents of someone with MS often feel in some way responsible. They will admit to a niggling fear that they may have passed on MS, although there's no medical evidence of a direct genetic link. They will also wonder if they failed to protect you from something in the environment that may have caused the disease.

It is understandable that they are concerned and wish to do what they can to help. They might be able to offer support in very practical ways, perhaps by listening, comforting, babysitting, assisting with household chores, gardening, or accompanying you to the shops and on trips. Their help may be invaluable if given sensitively and unobtrusively. As with your partner, much depends on the quality of your relationship with your parents before you were diagnosed, and how ready you are to initiate any changes that are needed.

There are some parents who find it difficult to accept MS, even when it is staring them in the face. It is as if they cannot accept that their child could ever have anything wrong. This attitude, which places a high priority on keeping the side up and achieving well, is one a child may also have shared unquestioningly. It is an attitude in which anything less than perfection is seen as failure. Unfortunately, this sort of attitude frequently stands in the way of coming to terms with MS.

It is not uncommon to discover that you are clinging on to values and opinions about illness and disability that you learnt at home as the norm, but that your new experience with MS demands you should confront. It is no help at all to persist in believing that having MS is somehow a sign of personal failure. Mavis's parents obviously felt this way about her, and were helpless to make any meaningful contact with their 40-year-old daughter. Like a little girl, she went through a phase of trying to please them and everyone else, as though to compensate for her MS. Far from getting her the understanding and support she so desperately needed, it only alienated her from her parents even more. The important factor for her and many others with a similar experience is that her previous relationship with her parents had never been that good, and she had always been the one who tried to compensate for the shortfall. As a child, she had never succeeded in getting the unconditional love she craved. Now that an MS diagnosis made her feel vulnerable, she needed that love even more, but her parents didn't know how to give it. The only practical solution was to keep a distance from them and for Mavis to get her support elsewhere. In order to do that, she needed to cut her ties and accept responsibility for herself. She had to learn that she had the right to make up her own mind and choose her own priorities, especially now she had MS.

There is a danger in some families with MS that the parents will come in and virtually take over. If that is what you (and your partner) want, then it is fine. If not, it is an invasion of your privacy, which you have every right to oppose.

It is hard to stand by when your own child is hurt: you want to remove the hurt and make it better again. Good parents will naturally feel protective and caring, and will look for ways to help. At the same time they will often experience helplessness too, and need guidance on how to relate appropriately to you.

Coping with friends

'You certainly know who your friends are when you've got MS,' say many people with the disease. You may suddenly discover that some of your friends have amazing depths of kindness, while others turn out to be the shallow, fair-weather sort. Some stick by you through thick and thin; others cool off and maintain a cordial distance for fear of getting more involved than they want to; and a few disappear fast.

The best friends are those who find out what you want and do not jump to conclusions. You have a responsibility to share with them such information about MS as will enable them to support you best. You also need to be

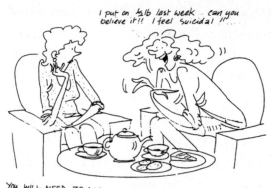

YOU WILL NEED TO DEAL WITH FRIENDS WHO TAKE ADVANTAGE OF THE FACT THAT YOU WILL ALWAYS BE AT HOME, SERVE DECENT TEA & COFFEE AND WILL LISTEN TO THEM

aware that friends will vary as to how much they actually want to know. A treasured few will let you pour your heart out, and you will soon learn to choose what and how much to share with whom. Friends can only take so much, and you need to respect their limits if you want to maintain contact. You will need to learn how to deal with friends who like to organize you, who blunder but mean well, who take advantage of the fact you may always be at home, serve decent tea or coffee, and will listen to them, and those who visit you out of sympathy, to do you a good turn. If you become unable to get about easily, you will probably find fewer opportunities to make and keep friendships going. At times MS will curtail social life. You may be the sort of person who fears speaking frankly in case you hurt someone's feelings, yet you sometimes need to say no to a visit or outing because it is just not one of your good days. In the end, communicating your needs so that you give your friends a chance to help meet them is one of the things that keeps the friendship going. It could be a new experience to get from a relationship as much as you give, and for a while it might feel lopsided. It is frequently friends, rather than close members of the family, who enable us to accept that MS does not diminish us but provides a new framework to live within.

Coping with your doctor

An MS diagnosis will mark the start of a new emphasis in your relationship with your doctor. In fact, it is a good time to check if you really have the right person – someone who is comfortable with you and your MS. The best doctor–patient relationship is one in which the patient is offered what he or she needs personally but in a strictly professional way. However, when a patient feels vulnerable – and this is common with an MS diagnosis – he or she may try to change the basis of the relationship and seek to make an ally of the doctor. The patient begins to expect more from the doctor than can be given professionally.

The first thing to be clear about is that no doctor, however good, will have all the answers. You can't demand more than a doctor can give, and you are certainly being completely unreasonable if you pester your doctor for detailed information about your *future* MS. What you may be doing is attacking the doctor with all the anger and resentment you have stored up because you don't want to have MS. Doctors are a common target for patients with chronic illnesses. You may storm, rant and rave, or plead, coax and cajole, but in the end you must accept that MS is a very variable disease and no two cases are the same. You are the one who is largely responsible for managing your MS, and you are wise to invite your doctor to work with you.

If your doctor could be completely honest, he would probably admit that he would rather not have any MS patients on his register. Doctors are trained to cure rather than treat. It is natural they should want their patients to get better – whether out of compassion, a desire to alleviate suffering, or a wish to be successful and see their skills work. You may not be aware that a GP rarely encounters someone with MS, so may know less about the disease than you do. However, GPs are always ready to find out how best to assist with symptom control. When specific difficulties arise, the GP normally refers you to a hospital neurology department or specialist centre, where you would see a neurologist and/or members of a multidisciplinary team, which would include an MS nurse, physiotherapist and occupational therapist. This team may call in other professionals as needed, such as a social worker, or specialist in urology, pain control or palliative care. Together with the neurologist, they work closely with you to determine the best package suited to your individual needs.

Your MS diagnosis presents a challenge to your GP. Doctors can offer you their full professional skills of treatment and management, but they know as well as you do that that won't always be enough. If they are blessed with the skills of good communication, effective counselling and insight, they will get close to meeting your needs as you battle to come to terms with MS. You will value your doctor for understanding that you sometimes need just to talk. You will spill out a catalogue of vague symptoms he or she can do little about, and have another go at winkling out new insights as to how you are really doing, knowing that there are no hard and fast answers. All the doctor can give is tender loving care, for you both know there is no cure. Value the GP who is able to give such care, and forgive the one who can't. The reason for not being able to may be to do with his or her own personality, with MS in particular, or because your personalities clash.

Doctors often feel inadequate or frustrated when faced with MS patients, which is hardly surprising when they have to face the brunt of their patients' emotional outbursts. Doctors must be careful not to take such attacks personally: they don't deserve your anger, but they hope its release will give you some relief afterwards. Few doctors have the time or skills to confront patients therapeutically and enable them to cope with the anger, bitterness, fear and sadness, and then move on to living well with MS. Some practices can refer MS patients to counsellors or psychiatric social workers for this kind of help. Alternatively, branches of the MS Society (see page 284) offer skilled support via trained voluntary workers, or within self-help groups.

There is a very real problem in coping with the hidden and subjective symptoms of MS. Both before and after diagnosis some GPs are sceptical about these, often labelling them incorrectly as 'neurotic' or 'hypochondriac'. What they need to realize is that you may experience so many of these symptoms that those you begin by describing may be chosen almost at random because they're the ones that have affected you most emotionally, or even because you have forgotten the others. It can be helpful to keep a list of what you want to share with your doctor. MS can make someone more prone than usual to forgetfulness. Doctors need to remind themselves that their MS patients do not necessarily know what weight to attach to their symptoms, and patiently wait to hear the whole list. Getting your doctor's support and understanding over fatigue, bizarre sensations, pain and visual problems is helpful because it confirms that these are recognized symptoms of MS, despite being sometimes attributed to other causes.

Tricky areas for doctors are giving advice about diets and alternative medicine. They have a responsibility to protect their patients from quackery and opportunists out for money. They are also concerned that false hopes of a cure are not raised when the treatment on offer defies all the laws of medicine and scientific reason. They would be unprofessional if they did not warn against unlikely cures. They understand the depression that results when a cure does not work. On the other hand, many doctors are happy to keep an interested eye on a patient who follows some diet or exercise regime as long as they are reasonably certain it will do no harm.

How to get the best from your doctor

- Be punctual.
- Be specific about why you are seeing him or her. A doctor needs to know if you have come for a chat, a prescription renewal, or specific help in order to give the appropriate response quickly.
- Explain clearly your physical symptoms, any reactions to medication and any other concerns – in that order.

- Take along a written list of questions you want to ask, and jot down the answers you are given, in case you forget.
- Follow the advice of your doctor. Ask questions if you don't understand or forget what is said.
- Be polite and generous as you share any information about yourself. You are your own expert in MS. Remember that your doctor cannot mind-read.
- Try not to become too familiar. Doctors are engaged in professional work, and are not there just because you need someone to chat to. They have a right to privacy away from the office.

Coping with work

MS has such a bad press that for some people the mere mention of it conjures up images of incapacity and paralysis. It is no wonder, then, that employers think twice before engaging someone with MS, and may try hard to ease out an existing employee who develops it. They need to know, for example, that paralysis is an exceptional symptom, and that most symptoms flare up and then either stabilize or die down again for a long period of time. Many people with MS can lead a perfectly normal working life, with little or no loss of working capacity. For those with mild or remitting forms of the disease (the most common types), the effects of MS are generally minimal for a long time.

Even when an employee is more seriously affected, employers can often negotiate what work can still be done, and how and where. Increasingly, people opt for flexitime, and with certain jobs, especially if there is Internet access, may split their time between home and workplace, a trend that may also suit people with MS.

From time to time you will need to assess the effect of your MS on the work you do, wherever you are based. As soon as MS begins to interfere in any way with your ability to work, you need to consider whether introducing changes will make it practical for you to continue working. Changes to work practices, allowing for longer breaks, or the use of special or adapted equipment, may need implementing. The greatest challenge lies in redeployment, especially from physically demanding and stressful types of work.

When to tell your employer

It is difficult to know when to tell your employer about your MS. You are not actually required to disclose your disability unless your symptoms constitute a health and safety risk, which can sometimes be the case with MS in certain work environments. On the other hand, deliberately evading the truth or dishonestly answering a medical question during an interview, for example, is a different matter, which may lead to disciplinary action, including dismissal. Disabled rights and responsibilities remain complex areas, even though discrimination against disabled people in employment has been outlawed in line with the European Union Council Directive of 2000. Direct discrimination, harassment or victimization on the basis of disability is a clear-cut legal issue. The intention is to stop disability being used as a reason for automatic redundancy

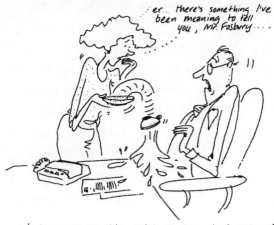

IT'S DIFFICULT TO KNOW WHEN TO TELL YOUR EMPLOYER ABOUT MS

or squeezing people out by pressurizing them into 'choosing' to leave because no other options are on offer. It is unlawful for employers to discriminate against disabled people when choosing someone for a job, or considering who to promote, dismiss or make redundant. These anti-discriminatory measures are intended to safeguard the rights of all with disability problems and ensure fair treatment. The onus is therefore on employers to make 'reasonable adjustments' in order to accommodate the particular needs of disabled people in their employment. It is generally wise for both employees and employers never to make assumptions, but rather seek expert advice. Similarly, employees with disabilities should demonstrate willingness to plan ahead – not easy to do, given the variability of MS.

Dealing with symptoms in the workplace

There is usually little point in rushing to change one's working lifestyle immediately after one or two relapses, unless you particularly want to escape work. It makes better sense to take off as much time as you need in order to recover as fully as possible from a relapse or bout of severe fatigue. Avoid rushing back to work earlier than your doctor advises, especially if you are still suffering markedly from MS symptoms. Safeguarding a good job that you enjoy and want to continue is so important to self-esteem and financial stability that you need to give yourself the best chance of continuing with it. However, as soon as MS begins to interfere in any way with your ability to work, you need to consider whether this is the time to introduce any changes that will enable you to carry on working more easily. Having to give up work completely is usually traumatic, even when it is also something of a relief. It involves a tremendous loss in terms of job satisfaction and personal identity.

If the symptoms you are currently experiencing are invisible, you may find it beneficial to explain to your employer that, though not obvious to anyone else, the symptoms are real and need to be addressed. You should suggest new ways of tackling your job or modifying conditions to make it easier for you to continue to work. If you hide behind invisible symptoms, you are not only multiplying stress and strain for yourself as you try to minimize the effect, but also leaving yourself open to being misunderstood. This happened to Gloria, who managed to land a temporary clerical desk job some months after giving up her permanent teaching job. Its part-time hours and routine work suited her as she didn't need to leave her desk very often. It soon became clear, though, that she too was expected to take her turn in fetching the drinks on a tray from the dispenser downstairs. She knew she'd have a problem managing the stairs and a full tray, so made various excuses to avoid the task. Soon it blew up into a confrontation. The others clearly thought she was acting a bit above herself, so to prove she wasn't, Gloria went and got the drinks. When her boss found her struggling up the stairs, precariously balancing a laden tray, he realized that something else was perhaps to blame. Once the MS problem was made known, a compromise could be reached and good relations were restored.

Thus, invisible symptoms can prove more difficult to cope with than visible ones, but can be resolved with careful management. For example, urgent and frequent urination becomes less of a problem if you can relocate near a toilet and your colleagues understand it's a common MS symptom. Similarly, fatigue that can sweep over you like a tidal wave so strong that you have to rest for a while can be coped with if your employers agree to your taking rest periods and provide somewhere suitable for you to lie down. Working flexitime, taking work home to finish, or going part time may prove more suitable.

It may be possible in an office-type job to make up for work left incomplete due to fatigue or eyesight problems when you have got back your normal energy. But that approach cannot be applied to manual work or if you just have to keep on the go, as in nursing, for instance. Heavy physical effort or intense mental strain day in and day out may even trigger a relapse or make symptoms worse. Sometimes it is possible to override or mask symptoms by sheer determination, but this works only in the short term. You find yourself getting through the week but collapsing exhausted at weekends, and getting through the day only to flop every evening. If work is a priority, you might accept this routine, even if it's a steep price to pay. But when the next day arrives before your energy reserves have been sufficiently topped up, you could find you are running yourself into the ground. This is when you need to reassess how many hours per week you can work and whether it's advisable to carry on doing that type of work. Physical work involving exertion or fine, coordinated movements of hand, leg and eye may have to be given up and alternative work considered. This is what Nigel did. He was an optician in his late fifties when diagnosed with MS. Although he could no longer manage to work as an optician, he felt sure he could now make a pipe-dream a reality. At home he equipped a workshop with wood-turning equipment, and from a much-loved hobby grew a small but successful and rewarding business.

Help is a two-way street

It is important not to become a limping liability at work. Apart from being a danger to yourself, you might be a safety hazard to others if you fall over, especially if there is equipment nearby. You might have to rethink your job so that you can limit how much you move about. Using a scooter or wheelchair may become a safer, quicker way of getting around – perhaps the only practical way. It will probably involve relocating to the ground floor, unless a lift is available. Access to your place of work will also have to be checked, and ramps, widened doorways, adapted toilets and specified parking provided. All employers are, in fact, required to make full access provision for disabled employees. Even if they would prefer the easier option of employing someone who is not disabled than catering for someone who is, it is a legal requirement to do so.

The fact that you can't rely on your walking might never interfere at all with your ability to perform your work well. If or when it becomes obvious to your work-mates that you have a physical disability, they will be challenged to accept that this need not debar you from work. Mary has discovered that because she is excellent at her job, her colleagues completely ignore the fact that her scooter has become her legs. To compensate for her disability, she has chosen to focus on doing a top-quality job, and that's working well for her.

In general, employers and some colleagues manage very well when they know what MS symptoms can occur, and are happy to adjust if you take a positive and inform-ative approach. Once they realize that symptoms normally fluctuate and disappear fast, they cope well enough.

Should you give up work?

Loss of employment has such a devastating effect that you will do best to stay at work as long as you want to. Most people need to work for their own personal satisfaction, as well as to remain financially independent. To be deprived of work is a blow that robs you of status, a regu-lar routine, and the knowledge that you are contributing to society. This is especially true if you are the bread-winner. Loss of a job results in diminished self-worth and a subsequent withdrawal from society. Men and women with MS, especially when the main income earners, find it very difficult being workless. Despite greater sexual equality in the workplace, men in particular report how gutted they are when MS stops them from working in their chosen occupation. All those who can no longer work but wish they could are likely to struggle with feelings of rejection or being distanced not only from their workmates but also their partner at home, who will have to take up the slack. As a consequence, the non-working partner with MS may feel doubly insecure.

Increasingly, people need to be better informed about the effects of MS on work. In Britain, the Department for Work and Pensions has set up the 'New Deal for Disabled People' specifically to support anyone who receives disability or health-related benefits. It operates through a network of job brokers experienced in working with people with health conditions or disabilities. They understand your situation and offer practical help in finding employment that you would like to do. This may involve offering extra training and support, plus help in overcoming mobility issues or lack of confidence. For contact information see page 291.

Coping with domestic responsibilities

It is relevant here to mention the chores that are a part of everyday life. Shopping, washing, cleaning and preparing meals all have to be done. Whether you are single, or have a partner or family, your MS might make this type of work difficult too. Mothers with MS who have young children to care for often find housework is more than they can manage with the reduced energy and the symptoms they are experiencing. It is hard to ask for and get the type of help you

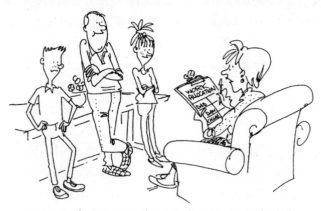

DURING A RELAPSE A MOTHER MAY BE FORCED TO LIMIT HER RUNNING OF THE HOME TO AN ORGANISING OR COORDINATING ROLE...

want, but remember that partners, relatives, neighbours and friends can be very supportive in practical ways. During a relapse, or when disability persists, a parent may be forced to limit her/his running of the home to an organizing or coordinating role. The physical chores are undertaken by others, including support from outside, if appropriate, but the parent uses practised expertise to help plan and budget whenever possible. This is an option that allows for a continuing valuable contribution to be made, although its less active nature might provoke some frustrations.

Social attitudes to sickness

A diagnosis of MS does not necessarily imply either sickness or disability. The frequent response of 'But you look so well!' indicates not only that looks belie a person's condition, at least at first glance, but also that with MS someone is clearly not sick in the conventional way.

Society tries to contain sickness by specifying certain conditions that the sick should fulfil in order to get rid of the illness so that once again, when recovered, they may resume their place. Unless you understand that society is full of unspoken assumptions and expectations we all automatically buy into, you may well feel affronted by the reactions of people towards your MS.

Society's first assumption is that the sick should be pronounced so by doctors, withdraw to an isolated position and give up social responsibilities until health is restored. Even if your sort of MS doesn't obviously affect your lifestyle, and you believe this rule does not apply to you, there will be some people who expect you to adopt a sickness role anyway. Frequently, though, the fluctuations of MS will result in your curtailing or opting out of some responsibilities at home, work and socially. If you are determined to hold a job down at all costs, you may not have the energy to garden or go to parties, so you will withdraw in order to maintain your priorities. This may become a more or less permanent way of life, so you need to make a determined effort if you want to counterbalance it with input that supports you and draws you back into contact with others.

Society's second expectation of the sick is that they should be taken care of. With MS this is applicable only during a relapse or when disability is severe. Apart from these times, you can maintain your independence and ask for what care you need when necessary.

The third assumption is that those who are sick should always want to get well. This probably causes the most irritation among those with MS. Of course you want to be well and never again be reminded of this chronic disease. If anyone could tell you exactly what to do to be well, you'd follow that advice like a shot, which is why so many so-called treatments and cures gain such a following. How well you are on an imaginary scale of nought to 10 can vary from less than one to more than eight in the space of a day, so you hesitate to commit yourself to saying how well you are feeling right now. With MS it is often wiser, and more within practical reach, to aim at improving your quality of life across the board than to expect a 100 per cent return to fitness.

The last expectation is that the sick should get the best medical advice and then follow it obediently. This is also of limited relevance, as MS requires a pooling of cooperative effort between doctors, other health-care professionals and yourself.

MS in a health-orientated society

When you have a chronic condition, such as MS, you may not class yourself as being in peak health, but neither can you necessarily claim that you are sick. You may experience spells of sickness, but the rest of the time you are either more or less aware of the fact that you have MS. You and those around you need to be clear as to whether having MS makes you a sick person or not. If it does, then you need to know how to react and what role is appropriate for you.

Approaches to MS

There seem to be three main reactions to being sick in a healthy society. Although you may not see yourself fitting any one of these patterns completely, you will probably recognize certain tendencies in yourself.

1. BELIEF IN THE MEDICAL PROFESSION

You may be the type who at the first sign of what may pass as a symptom, however mild, fleeting and unobtrusive, rushes to a doctor for diagnosis, care and cure. You are on your guard against potential illness and determined to avoid it. You have faith in the ability of doctors to remove ill health, and expect to receive treatment. When the cause of your health problem is MS you will soon be disillusioned because no doctor can give you specific advice on the cause, course, prognosis or treatment of your MS that will take it away. Doctors cannot know what is as yet unknowable. They have had to come to terms with this sort of frustration over and over again in each area of their medical training and practice. It is not unique to MS, but forms the barrier to knowledge in every branch of medical science. If you are potentially a doctor-dependent patient, believing that the medical profession should have all the answers, this is a hard reality to accept. If you cannot accept it, you will spend more time and energy on battling with doctors than on learning to live with MS.

2. BELIEF IN SELF-HELP

If you are the sort of person who takes total responsibility for yourself right from the start, you have probably been very aware of what has been going wrong in your body and have done all you can to improve your condition. You will have checked your diet, supplemented it with additional remedies, vitamins and minerals, and chosen to focus on what you know you can achieve, turning your back on any non-essential activities. You are in control, and have decided to do it your way. You are determined to preserve the outward signs of functioning healthily in a health-valuing society. And you have MS too. You may so value remaining part of society that you overlook the real effects your MS is having on you. By the time you are willing to admit to some health problem and see a doctor, your MS will have become visibly severe and you will probably have been pushed into seeking medical help by family, friends or colleagues. Self-reliant, you are used to driving yourself hard and determined to keep going, but you pay a heavy price. Yours is a tightrope of an existence in which you are maintaining the best lifestyle you can with your current health problems. It is precarious, but it means you avoid the sickness role and stay in the mainstream of society. Although you decide your own priorities, you can become so single-minded about keeping going at all costs that you neglect to ensure you have sufficient caring support from others. You need that balance.

3. BELIEF THAT ILLNESS DOESN'T EXIST

Maybe you are the sort of person who loves being part of society so much that you can never afford to be sick and take time off to recuperate. You will probably be aware of abnormal symptoms, but are unwilling to give up an active working and/or social life. You disregard the effects of MS by never adjusting your lifestyle, and going on to the point of total exhaustion and collapse. You believe that if you make any allowance for your MS, you are somehow giving in and failing. Yours is an all-or-nothing existence with high stakes. While the going is good, you can pretend MS does not exist, and enjoy the full swing of normal living. If ever your MS threatens to limit your activities and confine you away from the mainstream of society, you will struggle with the feeling that you have to shut yourself off from people. You are likely to need understanding help, and to be taught how to modify your reactions. With MS you have the right to be part of society, however highly that society values good health and feels discomfited by sickness.

Optimism versus pessimism

It has been suggested that optimism and pessimism are simply two different ways of handling anxiety. Optimists have naturally lower levels of anxiety than pessimists, and find that they can easily ignore the sort of situations that habitually stress those with a gloomier outlook.

Optimists see any problem as temporary, specific to a known cause, and nothing to do with themselves. They seem to possess a natural buoyancy that gives their bodies stamina to fight things off, probably including disease, and imparts mental courage to explore ways of over-coming difficulties. They avoid speculating over potential negative outcomes. They can laugh at themselves and their situation. It is not that optimists are immune to life's heavy blows, but they seem better equipped to ride them positively by looking on the bright side.

Riding bad situations doesn't satisfy dyed-in-the-wool pessimists, whose natural anxiety levels are higher than those of optimists. A pessimist is more likely to confront worries by thinking through all that could go wrong and developing strategies that have the potential to limit or ward off disaster. It's one way of taking control, a crucial and positive factor in handling stress well. Psychologically speaking, it's a more sophisticated approach because it involves learning how to face and tolerate negative feelings in order to achieve a desired outcome.

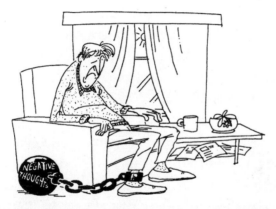

IF YOU ARE A DYED-IN-THE-WOOL PESSIMIST, YOU WILL LIMIT THE BODY'S REHABILITATION BY YOUR NEGATIVE THOUGHTS...

So which approach is best? When it comes to an uncontrollable condition, such as MS, a broad optimistic perspective will lighten the load considerably, but a willingness to analyse and tolerate negatives will result in developing workable coping strategies. It seems certain that we can all learn to think more positively, which has a beneficial effect on our health. Techniques of positive thinking teach us how to rewire our brains and stop chewing over bad experiences, a habit that contributes to depression. An example of positive thinking would be to focus on small experiences that bring us pleasure, a sense of achievement and feeling of well-being.

Exerting control

The issue of control is especially pertinent to diseases, such as MS, that strike at random and without warning. You are suddenly knocked off your feet – literally, as well as figuratively – and experience what it is like not to be in control of what is happening to you. This is very frightening, and your panic can spread to other areas of your life before it takes the time it needs to subside.

Once you begin to accept that you are still valuable as a person, even if your body does not always function in the way you would like, you begin to be in control of your own life and destiny again. Some people find a religious faith or philosophy of life helps them to achieve this. Others seek some sort of professional help from counsellors or therapists. Once in control, you experience freedom to grow as a person, looking for options, experimenting, always moving on. The disease may still be beyond your control in a medical sense, but you don't let it stifle who you are and what you want to do.

Some people use MS as a perfect excuse to control others and their environment. Since they can no longer control their lives as before, they concentrate all their controlling powers elsewhere. Ruth was a prime example of a controller. She sat in her chair and directed the household from there. She had everyone running at her beck and call. Her attention to detail was meticulous, and home-helps soon learnt to replace ornaments in *exactly* the same spots after dusting. Her controlling attitude towards family and friends gave her a sort of power to insist things be done her way, but not with a gentleness and warmth that attracted people to her or gave her happiness in living. While you have a right to take control of your own life, you have no right to trample over the feelings of others.

Having the right attitude

'It's your attitude that counts' is a statement that can get under your skin and itch. If pronounced like a challenge, it can sound rather damning. It seems to suggest that a simple change of attitude would rid us of any difficulty with MS and perhaps even remove it permanently.

MS gives you a fresh opportunity to rethink opinions, values and stances from a new vantage point. You will soon become aware of your attitude towards yourself, towards sickness, towards disability in general and MS in particular. The attitudes of people you know and society at large will come across loud and clear, and may surprise and shock you. It will take you time, frankness and courage to challenge any of these attitudes if you have to. Attitude can make a difference to physical, mental, emotional and spiritual well-being. You do not have to get it right all at once, but people with MS do need to get started as early as possible on developing the type of outlook that will help them live well with the disease. It is possible to win with MS and not to lose. It is never too late to look for options and make changes. This is the attitude that counts.

Accepting MS

Living well with MS means accepting that it has moved in with you. It's a bit like fitted furniture – so permanently there that in the end you do not notice it. MS may be something you cannot escape, but it need not be threatening. You do not have to welcome it like a friend, but you cannot ignore it either. MS must be accommodated. When you finally do so, you are entering a pact in which *you* become the expert on *your* MS. You will require information about the disease and support from many sources but you must take responsibility for yourself now and in the future. MS may scream, shout and throw tantrums, but it doesn't have to take over. You give it houseroom, but on your terms.

Reactions to disability

When MS symptoms interfere with your lifestyle you clearly face a problem with disability. It may be a disability that shows, and that you and others are already aware of. Or perhaps it is a hidden disability that causes some embarrassment, such as an incontinence problem (this can usually be managed quite discreetly with the right advice and protection). It may even be a disability that could be described as an exaggeration of what everyone feels from time to time – unutterable weariness to the point of tears.

People react to disability in various ways: hiding it or revealing all. You may be expert at brushing aside the genuine interest of others in your disability problem. Perhaps you are afraid of a flood of uncontrollable feelings sweeping over you once you start to talk about your symptoms and experience. You have to be with a safe and understanding person who asks at the right time and in the right way, or else it is just not worth the agony. Or you may keep quiet because you are uncomfortable or ashamed of your disability: it makes you feel different or even inferior. It is a documented fact that some people with a disability experience a distorted body image. They see themselves reshaped by the disability they are most aware of. It is like looking in a hall of mirrors at a funfair. They may also suffer from a sort of psychological distortion that makes them believe that disability confers a lesser status.

Some people, however, want to talk about their disabilities again and again. It is as though their experience and its impact on their lives are not quite real. Talking it out and being understood brings a tremendous relief. It helps them to accept, and gives comfort and courage to go on. For them, silence may impose an intolerable stress and lead to depression. Occasionally, people get stuck in rehearsing their story of living with disability and never move on. In this case, professional support can help them make a transition from being focused on their disability to living a positive life, albeit with a disability.

Another reaction is to fight MS disability doggedly, which has its plus points. You desperately cling on to what you know as normality. This can be positive if it means you continue to interact with other people, but it is often

an uphill struggle for all those affected by multiple sclerosis, which includes the entire circle of family and
friends. This reaction can also involve fighting against all
odds for equality within society. Recent legislation has
promoted a greater awareness of disabled rights, as seen
in the provision of disabled access to buildings. It is also
increasingly recognized that although people with disabilities may require support and care, they need not be
regarded as dependent. Indeed, in unique ways people
with disabilities may prove outstanding examples of living
with autonomy, self-reliance and independence. This is a
real challenge because MS fluctuates in its symptoms and
their severity. Add to this the MS fatigue factor and it's
hardly surprising that we often feel torn and experience
inner conflict. It's easy to find ourselves at one end of the
spectrum or the other – functioning well enough despite
disability, or struggling to cope. If the latter includes refus-
ing to learn to live with MS, there are serious problems
ahead. Some people hang on to the hope of a cure and
put their lives on hold while waiting for that day to arrive.
They exist, so blinkered to how MS limits their lifestyle
that they are unwilling to make changes that will accommodate their disease or disability. It's as if they expect
magically to step back into an MS-free life once a cure is
found.

The way you react to MS disability does not always
relate to how severe the disease appears to be. Some people
are devastated by minimal symptoms and handicap, while
others with severe disability take it all in their stride.
Responses are very individual and depend on personality, lifestyle, work and the support of others. Megan, who
has never been an outdoor type and whose legs are now

partially paralysed, does not hanker to roam the hills, but is quite comfortable relaxing with a book or watching TV. Her level of disability fits easily with her interests and preferences. Accommodating another MS disability, though, such as eyesight problems, would be quite a different matter for Megan. Andy, on the other hand, is an outdoor type, who mourns no longer being 'outward bound' or involved in rescue work. A desk job in the control room is poor compensation.

If a disability is obvious, everyone makes allowances for it, often giving you a wide berth or stepping in unnecessarily to help you out. Whenever you use a wheelchair, you take on a new role or identity, which others assume is permanent. Sam, with slow progressive MS, was a familiar and welcome figure locally over many years. His walking disability was relatively static, but confined him to an electric wheelchair from which he led an active social life, as well as being an ace organizer on behalf of all people with disability. A popular local mayor, with a similar type of MS, took a similarly positive approach. She not only remained active in local politics, but also held down a management post until retirement age. You have the right to choose how you want to come across. You can live a very fulfilling life despite disability.

In many ways it is actually more stressful to cope with invisible or partial disability because it's a strain for you and others around you never knowing what to expect next. It can also be a problem if your disability is not very obvious. In a restaurant, for example, move from a wheelchair into an ordinary chair and you will experience a change of attitude from those serving you. Get out of your wheelchair to stretch your aching muscles and walk around a bit and some people will look amazed, unaware that using a wheelchair might not be necessary all the time. Remain in your wheelchair and ask a shop assistant directly for what you want, or take out a credit card to pay the bill, and you will find some people visibly surprised that wheelchairs contain human beings who are lucid, intelligent, pleasant and even have a sense of humour. (By the way, driving a mobility scooter always scores highly – especially with children.) It is not easy to strike a balance between hiding your disability and accommodating it as part of your identity, but it can be done.

Choosing support

It is possible that you have never asked for support for yourself before. Perhaps you have been the one who has always supported others. If so, your biggest struggle in learning to live with MS may be allowing yourself the right to receive support.

It is best to get an early start and begin experimenting at once with ways of being supported on your terms in order to cope well with MS. You must be prepared to reject firmly but gently any moves by others to take over your life. You will also need to guard against becoming demanding and fussy, and instead focus on giving others the respect that you would enjoy. Take note of the ways in which you usually ask for support. Do you make demands as compensation for being dealt such a blow as MS? Do you manipulate others into doing things for you? Or is yours a genuine and straightforward request for support, fully allowing the person you ask the right to say no or suggest an alternative?

You may find yourself in the midst of a power struggle with potential supporters. If you are afraid of being taken over, fight to remain independent at all costs. Remember, you have the right to support – practical or otherwise – but you do not earn it at the expense of others thinking and deciding for you. This is as true for professional care as it is for care by family and friends. You remain responsible for yourself and should get what you want within the limits of your own choosing and the safeguards of the law.

It is particularly important to pay attention to needs beyond the practicalities of everyday life. Your social, creative, emotional, sexual, intellectual and spiritual needs also require attention. Everyone at some time deserves and benefits from such care, and there will be people around you to provide such support. They may be members of your family, friends or neighbours who spontaneously reach out to assure you that they care and will stand by regardless. Treasure them. Or they may be professional carers, whose warmth and personal concern shine through their work. Both groups form the basis of your support network. With their support you know you are fulfilled and living for a purpose.

Taking responsibility

Once you have accepted that MS is part of your life and that you will live well despite it, there are numerous things you can do to improve and safeguard your well-being.

Caring for yourself

- Make sure you live healthily, eating the best and healthiest food, taking short but regular periods of exercise, and enjoying all the relaxation and sleep you need.
- Cut out all non-essential activity that just wears you down in order to focus specifically on keeping your muscles working. Exercise, physiotherapy and/or yoga stimulate the use of alternative nerve pathways. Learn how to breathe properly.
- Move out of overdrive, decelerate and idle in 'neutral' whenever your body needs to. Strike a balance that suits you between doing too little and doing too much.
- Learn to pace yourself and be flexible.
- Ask for the help and support you need.
- Follow the medical advice you ask for, and try any reasonable medication, treatment or therapy offered.
- Find reasons for living by creating interests.
- Believe in yourself.

Caring about the way you feel

- Learn to become aware of your feelings and thoughts.
- Find ways of expressing how you feel without hurting others.
- Choose to have a positive outlook.
- Learn to face up to negative feelings and let them go.
- Avoid damaging emotional stress.
- Don't isolate yourself emotionally.
- Seek the support of others who understand.

Caring about the way you see life

- Become aware of the changes you are experiencing.
- Believe you can accommodate change in positive ways.
- Positive thinking can replace negative thinking.
- Learn how to deal with problems better by breaking them down into steps and setting a series of goals.
- Focus on the present and the future, not on comparing the past and the present.
- Prepare yourself to cope with the effects of MS on your life and relationships.
- Plan to substitute new activities for old ones that no longer work for you.
- Develop talents you have a use for *now*.
- Believe you will achieve a sense of peace and satisfaction when you come to accept the reality of your MS.
- Take hold of the support that a meaningful faith or philosophy of life offers.
- Continue to make choices.

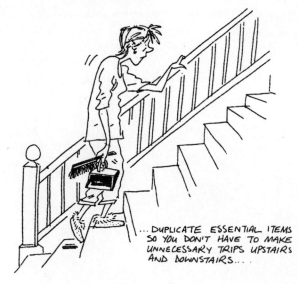

... DUPLICATE ESSENTIAL ITEMS SO YOU DON'T HAVE TO MAKE UNNECESSARY TRIPS UPSTAIRS AND DOWNSTAIRS....

Caring for the practicalities of life

- Get the difficult jobs done early in the day or whenever you have most energy.
- If you face a busy time ahead, plan opportunities to rest beforehand and afterwards.
- Use holidays to relax in.
- Check that the temperature suits you where you live and work.
- Try bathing in tepid or cool water.
- Keep stress and noise to a minimum.
- When you need to, use a stick, walker, wheelchair or scooter.
- Duplicate essential items so that you don't have to make unnecessary trips upstairs and downstairs.
- Vary what you do so that you don't strain one set of muscles.
- Take safety precautions, such as not picking up heavy objects that might affect your balance, or handling hot things if you are insensitive to heat, and never fill cups to the brim.

FOUR

Coping with the crises of MS

What turns a situation into a crisis? Is it events that create the crisis or the way we respond to them? We would suggest the latter. Some people will experience the so-called crises of MS written about in this chapter calmly, accepting each as simply another of life's challenges. Others may be devastated. Everyone has a different crisis threshold: some can take anything without batting an eyelid, while others crumple at the slightest thing out of the ordinary. We are all different.

A crisis throws you off balance. While it lasts, you are neither winning nor losing, but wavering in between. Although what some people call a crisis may not be one for others, that shouldn't make them distrust their own reactions. A crisis is a situation in which you feel vulnerable and at risk in some way. You are the only one who can decide what constitutes a crisis for you. The natural reaction to a crisis is to try to regain a feeling of ease. You experiment with various ways of coping, and when you find something that works, your balance is restored and the crisis consigned to history.

Some crises seem to escalate until they appear too big to handle. It's interesting to explore how this happens.

Initially people start off by coping with a crisis in the usual ways that have worked in the past. If it doesn't go away, they begin to feel tense and somewhat helpless. They usually discover that no one else has a ready-made solution to their crisis, so they are left to trial and error solutions that they have never used before. If none of these works, they feel extremely tense and very threatened. This then counts as an emergency and calls for drastic measures.

Some of these measures may have already been useful in coming to terms with MS. One approach is to change goals or aspirations. For example, instead of insisting on becoming a top footballer when you have a gammy MS leg that won't kick, you could choose a different career that doesn't depend for its success on that leg. Of course, that is easy to suggest, but it demands a real battle of relinquishment. No one gives up a dream without a lot of heartache. Another approach is to look at your altitude to MS. Is it fair to blame yourself for having the disease,

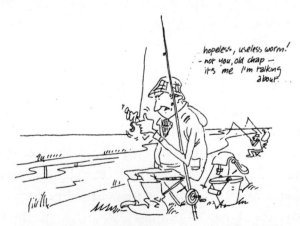

YOU MAY NEED TO CONSIDER HOW FAIR YOU ARE BEING WHEN YOU BLAME YOURSELF FOR NOT BEING ABLE TO DO SOMETHING LIKE TYING BAIT ON A FISH-HOOK

or even to blame MS itself? Learning to live within limitations is a tough assignment. We all get frustrated when we find it impossible to do something we've always managed to do before, such as tying bait on a fish-hook or threading a needle. Why not give yourself a break, grieve or get angry, and in the breathing space that follows allow yourself to find another solution to the problem? Often that solution will mean using another route, or involving another person. Of course, you could choose to ignore the problem – but just because a problem can't be solved as a whole doesn't mean that you should bury your head in the sand. Focus instead on solving just part of it.

Occasionally people become so tense over a crisis and so threatened that it all becomes too much and something has to snap. They may reach breaking point and collapse into deep depression, usually accompanied by a worsening of MS symptoms. This is the time for action by the medical profession, who will use a variety of means, such as tranquillizers, antidepressants, a stay in hospital, counselling, psychotherapy or psychiatric care, to help restore a state of balance.

The crisis process

A crisis, such as an accident, unemployment, death, an MS diagnosis or a new MS symptom, is a shock to the system. It is difficult to believe it's really going on and, in disbelief, you experience a sense of numbness.

After the shock and numbness you are likely to react in one of two ways – denial or outcry. Denying MS means shutting your ears to the facts given to you by doctors, ignoring what others say in confirmation of the diagnosis, and minimizing your own experience. You hear only what you want to hear, and search around for an alternative that gives some hope. Jeanette just couldn't cope with her MS diagnosis, and explained away her symptoms as arthritis to everyone she met. Only her husband knew the truth, and was ready to snap, especially when she kept on apologizing for her mobility problems, which he knew full well she couldn't do a thing about. He feared she was losing sight of reality. The mind goes round and round in circles, over the same old ground, but nothing changes. When your head is reeling, denial allows you time to put off taking stock. A delay in accepting the fact of MS is understandable, but remaining in a state of total denial means that your life goes on hold. You get frozen in time, with all your negative feelings buried alive.

Crying out against MS is a way of saying you feel victimized, it isn't fair and you don't deserve it – all of which are true. It is then a quick and easy step to blame others and seethe with anger. That may leave you feeling full of energy and buzzing around on a high, or you may hold on to those negative feelings of blame and anger, look visibly tense, and find your symptoms are aggravated.

After the denial or the outcry it is normal to experience a sense of loss. Losses deserve to be grieved for, as only then can a value be put on what you once had, and it becomes possible to move ahead to a fresh start. Loss is best gone through by allowing time and space for real crying. This helps release the tension. Finally you come to the point where you can see that what you are doing to yourself isn't helpful. At this point of exhaustion or panic comes the blessing of calm insight. All is not lost, and hope lies ahead.

It is now time to find out what is really going on, take a critical look at the situation and consider the options. This is when it helps to consider the opinions of others so that you have as much information as possible at your fingertips and can decide what to do for the best. It leaves you in the 'driving seat', still determining your course and not being taken over by others.

Some people find it too difficult to tackle a crisis, and refuse to go any further. They decide for many reasons, which they see as valid, that they are unable to take any action. It may be argued that they are overwhelmed by the difficulties, or that their worsening MS makes it impossible for them to do any more, but the reason for inaction lies mostly within themselves. They would need strengthened inner resources and extra special support and care from others to go any further, and they would also need to know how to accept and benefit from such help. They may seek refuge elsewhere instead, maybe in drink, drugs or self-pity, which compounds the crisis. It is a tragedy when someone cannot take steps to move out of the crisis, instead staying swallowed up in it, existing rather than living. To live well with MS it is necessary to go right through the crisis process until you find your way again – a new way to step out and on.

Common causes of crisis

As already established, stress does nobody any good – least of all those with MS. Unfortunately, stress is part of everyday life, so the best way to cope with it is to be prepared. Here we outline the most common causes of stress among those with MS and offer some ideas for dealing with them.

MS relapses, attacks and/or exacerbations

At diagnosis over 85 per cent of people with MS will be experiencing the relapsing-remitting form. In fact, having a relapse is what makes most people with MS contact the GP in the first place. Medically, any change in your MS condition in which new symptoms develop, old symptoms reappear, or disability occurs is called a relapse or exacerbation, provided the symptoms last more than 24 hours. In practice, people with MS often choose to distinguish the degrees of attack, characterizing them as major, minor or mini. Alternatively, they may refer to an exacerbation or setback, simply saying that their MS has got a bit worse recently but that they expect it to improve very soon. As always with MS, nothing is straightforward or the same for everyone.

EXPERIENCING RELAPSES

Relapses vary tremendously in type and severity, but they are always intrusive and never pass unnoticed. Some can be overwhelming in their impact, while others have a more 'contained', milder effect, manageable despite the discomfort and shock that accompanies them. During a relapse, MS symptoms can arrive or reappear quite quickly, sometimes within hours or over days, or they may build up slowly, tightening their grip inexorably. Not all symptoms are equally troubling, nor do they necessarily last long. They can last a relatively short time, or linger for weeks or many months.

If an exacerbation comes particularly suddenly, the person concerned will experience not only new symptoms or a recurrence of worsening old ones, but also a shock to the system. Some say that they can feel fine one minute, but the next they are aware of MS symptoms like a bolt from the blue. They may cope with resilience at the time, but experience an emotional reaction later as they adjust to the shock.

At other times there is a gradual build-up to a relapse, with symptoms surfacing so gradually that it takes a while to recognize what is actually going on. Often this is because you manage to block out symptoms. For example, numbness in a leg or hand may be uncomfortable, but you just get on with life and work regardless. During the build-up you may also experience problems in coming to terms with the fact that you do not feel so good. Evidence of the build-up remains highly subjective, so you might find yourself confused by its progress. You will probably also observe a gap between how you feel and what you want to do and what you really can accomplish feeling the way you do. Research into the common cold indicates that well before symptoms become apparent, the brain has already registered the start of the cold. For some people it seems to be like that with MS relapses, too. During the build-up it is common to be highly emotional. Some people find they cry a lot or feel unusually isolated from others and fearful that they are not acceptable.

Friends and relatives of people with MS need to

understand that this is quite common and part of a normal reaction. What people experiencing this desperately want at this time are tangible acceptance, love and support. They need supersensitive reassurance and understanding of how raw they feel. They want others to appreciate that they are acutely distressed. They do not need jollying out of it: at such times they can actually be unable to differentiate between what is meant seriously and what is a joke. Their mental processes may slow down too, and they may also feel depressed.

Most people find the symptoms that arise during a first relapse are temporary, and they recover fully from them. Typically, the symptoms include visual loss, double vision, weakness, unsteadiness and bladder problems. Although sensations such as tingling or numbness can happen to anyone for all sorts of reasons (or none in particular) and may have nothing to do with MS at all, they can also prove significant to a subsequent diagnosis of MS. The site of the damage determines what symptom develops. For example, optic neuritis occurs when there is inflammation in the nerve to the eye. This would probably be checked initially by an ophthalmologist, who might then suggest a neurological assessment. Weakness in the legs or loss of bladder control stems from spinal cord inflammation. Sometimes more than one site is affected. Fatigue and pain may be present, too. Although pain and fatigue are common MS symptoms, they are also associated with many other conditions, so are rarely considered to be diagnostic symptoms for MS. Certain transient symptoms that come and go over a minimum 24-hour period, such as a shock-like sensation when bending the neck, may also signal a relapse.

If you experience a very acute relapse, your GP may decide that you will benefit from being treated in hospital.

COPING WITH RELAPSES

During relapses people with MS may consciously work extra hard at keeping control of the situation. It is a characteristic way of trying to restore stability when life has become rocky and uncertain. If you can make sure that something will happen in a particular way or that someone will do what you want, you still feel in command of part of your life.

During an exacerbation people with MS may struggle with feelings of neediness. You may be the sort of person who normally attends to the needs of others and puts your own needs in the background. It is important to resolve this and find out how best to put yourself first for once. Often you need to release your feelings. A good howl with a stock of tissues can work wonders. You may want to be alone or very close to others, taking comfort from support and physical closeness.

It is the person with MS who is the expert when it comes to dealing with his or her own exacerbations. It is individual experience that counts – there is no need for anyone else to validate it. Although an exacerbation is an integral part of relapsing-remitting MS, it is unnecessary to give it more weight than it deserves. It will not go on for ever, and while it does you should try to feel positive about yourself, keeping your value as a person separate from the distorting experience of a relapse.

It is essential to find out how to cope with relapses. On the practical level you should shield yourself from getting overtired. The body needs to conserve energy to fight the exacerbation. Rest when necessary, but do not become immobile. Always aim to move about a little, and build this up gradually until a more normal state of mobility is reached, even if it is only now and again. Gentle exercise and massage may be helpful. If the main symptom is excessive fatigue, a person may feel he or she will never again have the strength to do more than just lie prone. However, the body *will* recover its strength, and as it does so in slow stages, make sure that normal activity begins as soon as possible.

It makes good sense to cancel appointments and any engagements that might cause particular strain. It is definitely best to refuse deadlines and not attempt to tackle problems, especially relationship ones. It is remarkable how effective letting yourself off the hook is. When you let go of pressures, you often find you feel restored quite quickly. Tom, a student with MS, suffered an exacerbation as he was working on a project with a deadline to meet. Forced to accept that he would not make the deadline, he put aside his work for a few days and rested. Within 24 hours he felt his symptoms easing, and after a few days was well enough to resume study. There is something healing about giving in to your body at the right time and being guided by what it says it needs during an exacerbation. It is a sort of pampering that is not indulgence but practical common sense.

WHAT ACTUALLY HAPPENS IN A RELAPSE

A relapse is thought to happen when the immune system damages a small part of the brain or spinal cord and that part becomes inflamed. This sort of inflammation within the central nervous system (CNS) brings with it the likelihood of damage to myelin and axons (see page 3). Such damage is usually repairable, and when that happens and remyelination occurs, you experience a welcome remission. However, if an axon is so badly damaged that it dies, no repair is possible. It is important to know that we can usually manage quite well enough, even though a lot of axons have been lost. There is a threshold beyond which further axon loss cannot be made good, and consequently symptoms and the level of function worsen. If it happens that the attacks repeatedly target one area of the CNS, the chances of complete recovery become less likely.

MEDICAL INTERVENTIONS

Neurologists agree that relapses need careful management and appropriate treatment. Relapses cause damage within the central nervous system and are bad news. The primary medical aim is therefore to reduce both the severity and frequency of relapses. In the long term neurologists would hope to eliminate relapses completely: any relapse would be regarded as a sign of failure.

Meanwhile, relapses are managed in various ways, the most promising being different drug treatments. A course of corticosteroids at high doses is normally prescribed for a short period of time to combat the effects of an acute relapse. Another option may be to start long-term treatment with one of the disease-modifying drugs (DMDs) now readily available, provided you meet specific criteria. Details of both of these therapies are given in the next chapter. Often bacterial infections, especially respiratory ones and those affecting the urinary tract, seem to be linked with relapses, so it is extremely important to get early treatment for them. If the time comes when new or worsening symptoms make it difficult for you to carry on your daily activities, you should ask to be referred to a specialized neuro-rehabilitation service or unit.

WHEN IT ISN'T REALLY A RELAPSE

Owing to the range of MS symptoms and sensations, it's easy to assume that whatever goes wrong in your body is the result of MS. It's therefore important to learn what the typical MS symptoms are and not to confuse them with any other aches, pains and discomfort. This applies not only to people with MS, but also to some medical professionals, who, if they are not really clued up on MS, may dismiss whatever ails you as 'just MS', when it could actually be a quite separate condition.

It is also important to learn that the reappearance of symptoms need not mean you are having a full-blown MS relapse. It will feel just like an attack because previous symptoms become aggravated temporarily, their effects lasting less than 24 hours. It does not result from new inflammation, but from certain triggers. One trigger is a rise in body temperature – perhaps you got over-heated from sunbathing, taking a hot bath, or exercising. Getting overtired is another trigger, as is fighting off an ailment, such as a cold, flu or urinary tract infection. So along with the reappearance of old symptoms, you may also experience fever or chilliness, nausea, vomiting or diarrhoea, or headaches, none of them MS symptoms. Episodes of this sort can happen very regularly, much more frequently than MS relapses, and are very wearing and distressing, but not for too long.

The reason for these episodes is that any minor rise in body temperature can slow down the way messages travel along the nerves. If certain nerves have previously suffered damage in the past, the slowing-down effect may result in old symptoms reappearing. Once your body cools down again, the symptoms usually disappear. They don't make your MS worse and are not life-threatening. Neither should they be used as an excuse to stop exercising regularly. Although exercise may cause a temporary blip, its overall benefits outweigh the temporary adjustment the body has to make. It always makes sense to let the body rest and recover after exercise. The key is to learn how to avoid getting overheated and overstretched by tuning into your body's energy levels and never pushing yourself beyond sensible limits. Although this is easy enough to say, it's impossible to achieve all the time with MS.

Some doctors suggest that MS can involve 'intermediate' relapses, which last longer than 24 hours and may not be linked with increased body temperature. As anyone with relapsing-remitting MS soon learns, there is no knowing what outcome to expect when symptoms familiar or strange start to intrude. It really helps to learn not to panic, and to find ways of 'riding' through all sorts of relapses for at least 24 hours. Our bodies may take a beating with MS, but we don't need to add to it by getting worked up. Keep calm and respond to the distress with sensitivity and gentleness. Take time to ease up and relax as far as possible, and only then decide if you need to seek medical intervention.

Twilight zones of MS

People with MS often talk about feelings and experiences to do with MS that are personal and subjective. They are not mentioned in texts on MS, but deserve to be given an airing. For want of a better expression, I call them 'twilight zones'. These elusive experiences, often difficult to define, may be characterized as transitory setbacks, slow-downs and low times.

EXPERIENCING A 'TWILIGHT'

The stark reality of twilight zones is that a lot is going on, and not only on one level. It is easy enough to focus on physical symptoms, or emotional reactions, or psychological musings, or events, places, people, diets, allergies and the like, and to disregard the totality of the experience. All these factors are part of a complex interrelationship. This is when you can lose sight of who you are, although you may still have some control and are not being taken over completely. You still feel some vestige of yourself – that you are a real, whole person.

You may feel that your energy is gone, that you do not know where feelings begin and end, and be uncertain about what pain is linked to which sensation. You doubt the provability of any particular symptom, and wonder if you are somehow imagining the strange jumbling of sensations, thoughts and feelings. Now is the time to relax and accept that this is another of the faces of MS. It is a most misunderstood phase, disputed even by some doctors, family members and friends. This is hardly surprising, for those with MS have often spent hours of internal dialogue, disputing with themselves whether what is happening is real. To cope you must accept that it is very real. In practical terms, if you have MS, you need to give yourself space and time to relax and soak up positive experiences. You should build in regular slots when you can rest as much as you need to and, as far as possible, do only what you want to achieve during this specific twilight.

AFTER THE TWILIGHT

What happens if you do not rest? You might get away with it this time, and even the next. By sheer will-power and determination, putting yourself into 'overdrive', you might talk yourself out of it or through it. Although you might succeed in pushing it out of mind and out of sight, it will have left its mark. Repeated setbacks similarly dealt with eventually have to be reckoned with.

The crunch comes when you are overwhelmed and suffer a severe relapse. All you can do is give in. You are an invalid again and it is obvious to everyone. The clear loss of energy and inability to manage everyday life indicate without doubt that you are struggling. Now you are faced with a slower, uphill fight to regain your strength.

Some people with MS deliberately choose this option as a coping mechanism. It buys what can be called 'legitimate space'. Everyone around has to admit that the person concerned has MS and is incapacitated by it. It is, however, an unhealthy way of coping because everyone suffers. It causes disgruntlement and strains relationships. However, there was a time, during the 'twilight zone' experience that preceded the relapse, when a warning was given. There was a chance at that point to salvage something and take action to ease the situation. Maybe even the relapse itself could have been prevented. So much is learnt in retrospect. The real challenge is discovering what patterns emerge from your own experience of the disease and how to use that knowledge beneficially in the future.

Fatigue

Have you ever started to tell someone just how unwell you have been only to be cut short by 'But you look so good'? The fact that you felt exhausted, together with all the niggling symptoms you were noticing and wanted to share, was brushed aside as apparently untrue. How can you look so good when you feel so rotten and wrung out? It can take a while to register externally what your body is telling you loud and clear inside – that it is profoundly tired by MS, a symptom known as fatigue. By the time you actually look fatigued, you have usually gone far beyond your limits. Fatigue is typically described as a chronic symptom, but that doesn't mean it can't become acute. If you become totally wrung out and incapacitated by fatigue, you are facing a crisis situation.

Fatigue probably affects up to 85 per cent of people with MS, so must count as a major symptom, but one that is hard to verify objectively. It is relatively easy to see if someone has any paralysis or tremor, or to spot eyesight problems. Fatigue is not identifiable or measurable in the same way. It is an all-pervasive symptom, an integral part of the disease and hard to understand, especially as MS fatigue is experienced slightly differently by everyone.

Sometimes it's just a passing symptom, but some people find fatigue settles in as a chronic condition. For many it's primarily about exhausting tiredness that overwhelms and curtails everyday living to a minimal level. It usually aggravates other symptoms, such as visual disturbance, impairs cognitive functions, such as memory and concentration, interferes with mobility and increases muscular spasms. Fatigue can be present in all phases of MS: in fact, it's often a first symptom that may go undiagnosed. It certainly makes a big impact on your quality of life.

Everyone knows what it's like to be tired ordinarily; indeed, tiredness can be a significant problem that leads people to consult their GPs. However, MS fatigue is more than ordinary tiredness. It's not that healthy feeling you get after a good day's work or a strenuous game of squash. It's profound and debilitating, but you may only realize this when it lifts. It can hit you suddenly and dramatically, as if a plug has been taken out and all your energy has drained away – you are zapped. Or it can creep up on you imperceptibly and you find yourself slowing down, dragging along with no push left. Everything is so much more of an effort. Most of the time fatigue is tolerable, simply a nagging unease and lack of bounce. At its worst, it resembles a bad dose of flu without the cold symptoms, and verges on a semiconscious state.

It is important to be aware of the differences between normal tiredness and fatigue. It is normal to be tired and ready to rest at the end of a day when you have overworked or not had enough sleep – a clear case of cause and effect. MS fatigue happens faster, lingers longer and takes longer to recover from. A few nights' good sleep will not necessarily do the trick. It appears to be primarily a neurological tiredness, with a physical cause, a result of damage to specific nerve fibres in certain parts of the brain – the basal ganglia and the thalamus – which are also involved in planning and coordination. In MS this fatigue slows down normal reactions. The extent of the tiredness, often called lassitude, bears no relationship at all to what you have been doing. The fatigue just appears for no good reason.

This particular symptom is not unique to multiple sclerosis: it is common in other diseases of the central nervous system, especially Parkinson's. Typically, there is a decrease in absolute physical strength. For example, the motor nerves are likely to be affected so that your muscles feel heavy and weak. Or after a short time using any given set of muscles, they tend to seize up – a 'short-circuiting' fatigue. You are likely to experience poor co-ordination, shakiness and exaggerated or inverted reflexes. The sensory nerves are affected too. Often people with MS become fatigued because they are over-sensitive to heat. This may be because of a rise in body temperature, or result from an external trigger, such as hot weather, a hot bath or hot food. Eyesight can become blurred, the speech slurred, hearing and the senses of taste and smell dulled. The sense of touch can be impaired and accompanied by tingling or numbness. Vertigo can become troublesome.

TRIGGER FACTORS

Certain triggers for tiredness affect everyone to a certain degree, and most people take them in their stride. However, when the body is in a borderline state, as is often the case with MS, those same triggers can have a more marked and negative effect. They include doing too much, a disturbed night's sleep, fighting off an infection, such as a heavy cold, heat, smoking, drinking, overeating, taking certain medications that have drowsiness as a side effect, feeling depressed or engaging in any activity for too long without a break. For example, it is normal for body temperature to fluctuate during the day and reach a peak in the afternoon. But in the person with MS a rise in body temperature can be enough to trigger a sense of deep fatigue. It helps to find out what your ebb times are so that you do not plan anything demanding then. Pam regularly rests straight after lunch to get over her tired spot in the day, and finds that doing so gives her the energy to cope with the children when they get home from school. Fatigue can also be a symptom of fighting off infection. Raj has noticed that he rarely comes down with the bugs that lay his colleagues off sick, but he often feels very tired at that time, presumably because his body is fighting off infection.

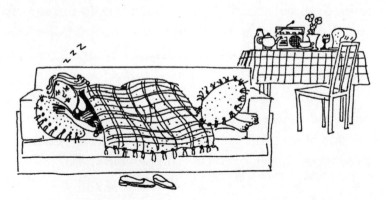

PAM REGULARLY RESTS STRAIGHT AFTER LUNCH TO GET OVER HER TIRED SPOT IN THE DAY...

Given that fatigue has different causes, the approaches to managing it will vary. Any central nervous system damage results in more energy than normal being used up. The result is increased weakness and lack of coordination. It really does not take much to tire the CNS. A knock-on effect is that some muscles have to work extra hard to compensate for the weakened ones, so they get tired faster. This, combined with the reduced energy output of MS, means that normal muscle fatigue is felt more often and more quickly. This helps explain why you may look well, initially feel well, and start off doing something well only then to have to stop suddenly because of fatigue.

PSYCHOLOGICAL FACTORS

It is difficult to assess from a clinical point of view what actually causes fatigue, what is a physical MS symptom, a reaction to having MS, and/or a depressive or anxiety state. Fatigue is bound to have a depressive effect and result in some anxiety. This is in addition to the anxiety and depression that frequently accompany MS anyway and that are expressed in feelings of tiredness, lack of energy and heaviness. The effect is therefore doubled. It is no wonder that some people with MS fatigue are at first misdiagnosed as neurotic. Doctors find that some patients hide or fail to identify the existence of fatigue as an MS symptom in contrast to others who appear to over-react to fatigue and exaggerate their symptoms, often dramatizing them in an emotional way. Faced with such different reactions, it is understandable that doctors may find it difficult to gauge how real a symptom fatigue is for any particular patient. What GPs understand from experience is that the way patients perceive their tiredness seems to contribute to the way it develops. Our attitudes towards tiredness or any other body ailment do make a difference. For example, perfectionists report higher levels of fatigue and worry.

Whatever the trigger, MS fatigue appears like a psychological reaction rather than the physical one it really is. Fatigue does, however, have a pronounced effect on symptoms, which well up and show themselves only when you are tired. You may feel you are heading for a relapse, but these old symptoms are merely temporary. Also common and temporary is a slight personality change. You feel out of step with yourself and under the weather.

WORKING AROUND FATIGUE

Fatigue is not harmful so long as you work around it rather than fight it. Struggling to keep going at all costs is counterproductive. If you become fatigued for a long period of time and do not get enough sleep and rest, you run the risk of serious physical harm, which takes a long time to reverse. Sometimes you have to fight yourself first before allowing yourself to rest as you know you need to. It's a fight against pride, needing to be always in control and forcing the issue.

Life becomes easier by learning to recognize fatigue before it catches up with you. Of course, it's not always possible, but it's well worth a try. It is important to keep physically fit, eat healthily and give up smoking. What helps most is pacing and planning the day, with rest and relaxation periods built in. Burning the candle at both ends just does not work with MS. In fact, one of the most helpful tips is to build in breaks, even very short ones of a few minutes, so that jobs and activities are done in stages, not in one concentrated go. It certainly helps to learn some techniques for managing MS. It is also useful to modify and simplify your lifestyle and home to meet your needs. Learning how to prioritize tasks is vital. Put off what you don't need to do today or ever again. Get the help and support you need to maintain your quality of life. Learn how to request it courteously and, whenever possible, in advance of a crisis situation. There is no point in dragging on endlessly with chronic fatigue. It's better to face the fact square-on and shed burdens earlier rather than later. In particular, being able to share all this with someone who accepts the truth of MS helps so much. It relieves a lot of tension and feels very supportive.

Fatigue has at last become recognized as a serious symptom of MS that needs a multidisciplinary approach. For example, physiotherapists are skilled at strengthening, stretching and relaxing muscles, which improves movement and circulation, while occupational therapists can teach you new ways of carrying out daily tasks in energy-efficient ways. People with MS may have to be firm about what they know they can and cannot do on any given day because of fatigue, and not allow themselves to be bullied into doing more than they should. Family and friends also need to have explained to them how necessary it is for those with MS to conserve their energy and spend it on whatever they decide are priorities. Ideally, that regularly includes fun and pleasure.

Impaired mobility

At some time or other people with MS are likely to experience difficulty in using their legs and arms. Obviously, there must be something wrong when, for example, you find it increasingly difficult to walk, moving first from using a stick to a frame, then needing a wheelchair for trips outside the house, and finally for permanent use indoors as well. This spells a crisis because of the dramatic effect loss of mobility has on the body and consequently on lifestyle generally. Not being able to walk well or use your arms normally feels wrong and is alarming to yourself and others. It immediately threatens to compromise your previous independence. Prolonged loss of mobility is generally associated with the progressive stages of MS. What is not known is how temporary mobility problems might be and how much they might interfere with life. It works well to assume that they are not going to last, and

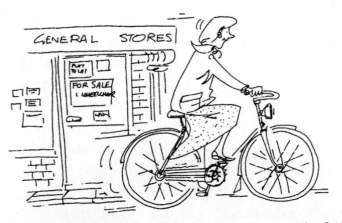

EDITH NEEDED TO USE A STICK, THEN A WHEELCHAIR MORE OR LESS PERMANENTLY FOR SOME YEARS TODAY, HOWEVER, SHE WALKS NORMALLY AND HAS TAKEN UP CYCLING AGAIN...

meanwhile to make use of whatever help is needed to get around more easily. Edith needed to use a stick and then a wheelchair more or less permanently for some years. Today, however, she walks normally and has taken up cycling again. Some time ago she wrote to cancel the mobility allowance she had been granted for the rest of her working life because her walking problems had been so severe. She no longer needed it. Impaired mobility may not actually reflect any deterioration in someone's MS, but is rather a sign of where a lesion is located and evidence of a relapse.

BALANCE AND COORDINATION

Mobility is affected by a number of different factors, which include problems of balance and coordination, tremor and spasticity. It is helpful to be aware of what can hinder smooth, spontaneous movement.

A particular type of balance problem, often referred to as *vertigo*, has a devastating effect on the way someone normally gets around. It can be fleeting or last for several weeks. It is a sort of dizziness in which the ground can seem to pitch, roll and toss like a boat in a storm. Some people also feel nauseous, and may even get to the point of vomiting. Trying to walk with this going on is distressing and energy-consuming. Also, it is not always obvious to other people why you are experiencing difficulty. A stick can be useful to give balance and warn others. Vertigo is normally accompanied by weakness and fatigue, and can persist even when you are not trying to move about. If very severe, even lying flat and not moving at all does not take it away. In such cases, all that can be done is to rest and see if any type of medication helps. Fortunately, vertigo is usually only mildly bothersome and clears up quite quickly.

Lack of normal coordination in the legs, arms or both has a clear effect on the ability to move normally. At times it can become a source of embarrassment, for poorly co-ordinated legs produce a staggering gait (*ataxia*) that any drunkard would be proud of. It was the sort of walking problem Kate was struggling with, her legs crossing in front of each other and going their own wilful way. It was impor-tant to her that she saw her young daughter to and from school each day, but hard to manage with ataxia. She had so far hidden her diagnosis from her neighbours and the other mothers at the school gate, but she could not hide the evidence of her MS walk. Only when she learnt that people thought she had taken to drink did she decide to share the fact that she actually had MS. She was warmed by the support and genuine concern she received. Practical help came her way, as others offered to share in fetching her daughter from school when necessary.

Sometimes it is the arms rather than the legs that are affected. Weakness in the arms is particularly devastating because we rely so much on their strength and coordin-ated movements, and the dexterity of our fingers. For example, you reach out to take or return something and miss, which can be expensive in terms of broken crockery and very frustrating. An associated problem is when the hand may begin to shake as soon as you intend to carry out any action. Called an *intention tremor*, this symptom results from interference along the nerve pathway.

Tremor can also affect the legs, trunk and head. Seventy-five per cent of people with MS experience the way it interferes with daily activities at some stage. Mild tremor is wobbly and unbalanced movement, which responds to physiotherapy on the affected muscles. Severe tremor, with its unpredictable movements, is best treated on an individual basis.

SPASTICITY

Coordination disturbances and spasticity tend to occur simultaneously in MS. Spasticity, a term that covers the symptoms of stiffness and spasm, is a predominant motor disturbance of MS, and it can sometimes become severe. Spasticity is high in certain groups of muscles and forms an abnormal pattern of movement. If a health professional attempts to move the limb of a person with MS who is trying to relax, there may be a significant resistance from the muscle(s). In order to move effortlessly, one set of muscles will contract while another relaxes. If the muscles all contract at the same time, the result is stiffness and/or spasm, which restricts movement. Spasticity is actually an overenthusiastic response to a stretch of the muscle. As a result, everyday activities, such as walking, sitting in a chair, eating, turning over in bed, and caring for yourself, can become difficult. Spasticity can also affect sexual activities, your mood and feeling of well-being. The effects may be quite mild and happen only occasionally, or severe and longer lasting. They usually vary from day to day or during the day.

Spasticity can be aggravated by other factors, even a full bladder or constipation. Other common triggers include infections and pain, such as toothache or an ingrown toenail, pressure sores, poor posture and even changes in humidity or temperature.

Understandably, coping with spasticity is more than a physical challenge. It has the potential to impact on your way of life negatively, threatening your ability to care for yourself the way you used to and still want to. Living with spasticity evokes a strong emotional response: feeling frustrated and helpless is inevitable if you can no longer manage the everyday things the way you used to do without thinking. Although it is often possible to allocate tasks to others if you can't do them, it hits hard if your contact with the outside world becomes curtailed.

Stiffness in the limbs is a common symptom that interferes with activities that demand coordination or fine movements. It is particularly hard to cope with if your hands and fingers are affected: you quickly discover how many movements your hands normally make in a day. Often it is a stiffness that gets worse with movement. Gillian knows that on a good day her stiff legs will take her to the local shops and back with the help of a stick. It is worth the struggle for the friendly chat and the sense of achievement on arriving back home with a few purchases. On not so good days her legs seize up by the time she has reached the end of her road, and it is all she can do to get back to the house.

Stiffness is fatiguing and disabling and it is not worth forcing the body to achieve what it refuses to do. Instead, let it ease up and coax it back into movement when it is ready. Some of the drugs that are very effective against spasticity also have the side effect of increasing weakness, so that the legs seem to turn to rubber. The medication enables suppleness to return to the limbs but they lose their strength to support. The one advantage of a stiff leg, provided it isn't also weak, is that it can sometimes be used as a prop and pivot.

Spasms are uncontrollable and usually very painful contractions of muscles. They leave you feeling wrung out and add to fatigue. They can happen day or night. They can sometimes be set off by apparently minor movements, like coughing, sneezing, hiccoughs or even laughing. Two particular types of spasm can become troublesome with MS.

• Extensor spasms can occur when attempting to make a movement. Both legs shoot out straight and are then difficult or impossible to bend. It looks and feels alarming, but is seldom painful. Sometimes bending the neck so that the chin moves towards the chest can terminate the spasm. Extensor spasms often seem to occur at night, and rudely awaken you – and your partner. Seeking a physiotherapist's advice on sleeping positions can help here.

• Flexor spasms are usually a later development, and are most often experienced by those in a chronic progressive stage of MS. The muscles involved here are those that bend the leg at the knee and hip joints. If you are on your feet at the time, the result of a flexor spasm is that you fall over. They are more painful and can happen even when you are sitting or lying down. Any infection of the bladder or any sore place on the legs seems to aggravate them. The drug Baclofen (Lioresal) is of particular use, as it acts specifically to dampen down any abnormally active reflexes.

In the case of severe disability, more permanent measures, such as nerve-end blocking or surgical procedures, may be needed so that you can sit or lie in comfort. The great fear with impaired mobility is always that it marks the start of a progressive stage that will catapult the sufferer into irreversible disablement. Such stages are characterized by a progressive decline in neurological function over a period of more than six months. They are rare early on, but may develop after several years of MS. It seems that the prognosis is most favourable if MS follows a benign course for the first 10 years.

As spasticity varies in its symptoms and their severity, treatment will be offered from a range of practitioners and health specialists, starting with the GP, and moving on to the neurologist, rehabilitation and/or pain specialists, physiotherapist and occupational therapist, nurse and carer. Physiotherapy on a regular basis is thought to be most effective, as it focuses on keeping the limbs working as normally as possible, reducing the severity of muscle spasms and helping to prevent contractures, which is when weak, paralysed or unused muscles start becoming permanently shortened. Quick and simple daily exercises are beneficial, as is the correct posture in a chair or bed because it avoids the development of pressure sores and spasm. One tip to 'break' a spasm is to apply pressure on the affected limb, but beware: this is the only intervention to use, as fighting spasm in any other way only causes more pain.

In addition, certain drugs prevent or lessen spastic symptoms. Some, such as Baclofen (Lioresal), Tizanidine hydrochloride (Zanaflex) and the now little-used Diazepam (Valium) target the spinal cord in order to reduce the excessive activity that leads to spasticity.

Alternatively, Dantrolene (Dantrium) works directly on the muscles and reduces contractions.

WHEN WALKING FAILS

Not being able to rely on your own two legs to get you around may be reason to panic, but it is more constructive to consider alternative means of getting about. Sylvia recalls the time when the reality of her limited ability to walk hit her really hard. She was just beginning to feel that she was walking more steadily and picking up speed, when one day a little old lady, clearly walking slowly and with some difficulty herself, not only caught her up but overtook her and disappeared round the corner. She felt devastated and sobbed when she got home. It just wasn't fair. For Sylvia it was a true crisis situation, and she had to think long and hard about resolving it.

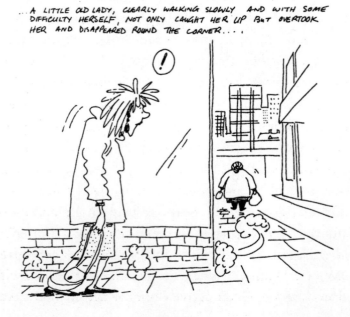

...A LITTLE OLD LADY, CLEARLY WALKING SLOWLY AND WITH SOME DIFFICULTY HERSELF, NOT ONLY CAUGHT HER UP BUT OVERTOOK HER AND DISAPPEARED ROUND THE CORNER....

When it comes to mobility or lack of it, the choice is limited: discover new ways of staying mobile, remain confined and isolated at home, or depend on others. The first option is preferable in theory, but in practice it is a tough option to follow. There are obvious reasons why people would rather not use a stick, a walking frame, scooter or wheelchair. These are the badges of disability we would all rather avoid. Society expects you to be either able-bodied or disabled, ignoring the reality of a middle ground. This needs confronting because life is full of experiences never faced before that each individual must be helped to cope with. A stick enables you to keep your balance and acts as a warning sign that you may move slowly. A scooter or wheelchair enables someone who cannot walk easily to stay mobile. Using a blue badge enables you to park your car near the shops. Knowing when to make use of these mobility aids is difficult and another potential MS crisis.

Take the prospect of using a wheelchair. It may so petrify you that you would rather stagger yourself to a standstill and collapse in a heap first. You may even be encouraged by doctors to keep out of a wheelchair as long as possible. They have a point because certainly there will always be a minority who use a wheelchair before they really need one and never plan to get out of it again. It is also conceivably a way to achieve the easy life, or a signal that they have given up the fight. If people lack power and ease in their lives to the extent that sitting in a wheelchair is going to resolve it, they may need counselling help. Telling them to use a wheelchair only as a last resort is not offering help where it is needed. Most people with MS need to be encouraged to use a wheelchair the way they use sunglasses – when the conditions really demand it. Using a wheelchair when it is absolutely necessary conserves energy and combats fatigue. Few parents would insist that their toddler, having once learnt to walk a few steps, should never again jump back into his pushchair. It makes sense to him and his parents to do so when he's tired or they need to get somewhere in a hurry.

Wheelchairs come in a more attractive range of colours, styles and sizes these days. They are either electrically powered, propelled by hand by the user, or pushed by someone else. It is less easy to be independent when you rely on another person to do the pushing. However, you need to have some strength and flexibility in your hands to control a wheelchair, even an electric one. It is usually worth persevering, though, for the thrill of independence you experience from being able to get around on your own. Scooters are an even more attractive alternative, as they are easily manoeuvrable and create a stir with the kids, who hang around hoping you will get off and give them a go. Battery cars are popular with some too, as they can be driven on the road and will travel many miles before they need recharging. The more people with MS and other disabilities make use of and have fun with their wheelchairs, scooters and the like, the sooner other people will be forced to change their preconceptions. Sitting in a scooter or wheelchair does not actually change you into a moron, and it is high time that that misconception was challenged.

If mobility problems are to do with balance and coordination rather than spasticity, a stick or some other type of support may be enough. If you have young children, you will find pushing a pram or pushchair can help to steady your balance. Shopping trolleys of the right kind can be a walking aid too. A walking frame is often very useful; some have wheels attached, and a basket or resting seat attachment.

Without doubt, a car is the most convenient way to keep mobile where longer distances are involved. You may find it easier to drive an automatic car, or have the hand controls and pedals adapted. The adaptation process is straightforward, and even automatic cars can be adapted for left-foot acceleration. If you are unable to walk, or walk only with great difficulty, you may qualify for the Mobility Component of the Disability Living Allowance. There is also a Motability Scheme, which enables you to use your Mobility Allowance to purchase and run a car. The blue badge scheme is invaluable because it allows you to use parking spaces designated for the disabled, and gives the right to park for a limited time where no other vehicles can. The local offices of the Department of Health and Social Security will be able to provide you with details of these schemes.

Using public transport becomes tricky when you have a problem walking and keeping your balance. You have to be somewhat agile to enter or leave a bus or railway carriage. However, there are likely to be some 'low-loader' buses in your locality, which makes getting around much easier, especially for people in wheelchairs. If you have a disability that does not show, it is worth carrying a stick to make it obvious, otherwise you can get jerked off your feet because the driver does not realize he should give you time to sit down before he pulls away. Coach operators and British Rail are generally very obliging and make special provision if you have a mobility problem. You need to warn them in advance so that they have time to make arrangements. The same is true when travelling by air. If you contact the airline ahead of time, they will make sure you and any escort get into your seats with a minimum of difficulty.

Pain

'At least you don't get pain with MS' is one of those infuriatingly inaccurate statements that too many people trot out as fact. When you reply that you do suffer pain, your answer is largely dismissed. It feels as if the person talking to you is saying that having MS is quite enough, and pain on top of it is taking things a bit far. (Of course, when you do have pain with MS, it does feel as if you're doing extra penance.) It is puzzling that for so long popular opinion, even among health professionals, refused to believe that MS could be painful. Until recently, medical textbooks also ignored the reality of pain occurring with MS. Now, however, the accumulation of evidence that many, but not all, people with MS experience pain has resulted in better pain management.

The pain spectrum runs from minor aches and twinges common to most people through to MS revolving around pain. Pain relief clinics report that persistent pain in MS is one of the trickiest problems to deal with because the cause of pain is difficult to diagnose and treat at the best of times, and particularly so if MS is involved.

Pain is very real and very frightening to the person who is suffering it. Accepted as a sign that something is wrong, physically or emotionally, pain is generally taken as a serious warning. However, as far as MS is concerned, pain does not necessarily indicate a worsening of the disease. It may have nothing to do with MS at all, and even if it does, it need not spell deterioration. Primary pain associated with MS is a direct result of MS lesions impacting on the central nervous system, and thus termed neurogenic or neuropathic, while secondary pain is referred to as musculoskeletal.

PRIMARY MS PAIN

There are many different types of primary pain, including pins and needles anywhere, tingling, shivering sensations, weird burning pains, as if you are on fire, feelings of pressure, and heightened sensitivity to touch on isolated tender patches of the skin or teeth. These pains cover the whole spectrum from aching, throbbing, stabbing, shooting and gnawing to 'electric shock' sensations. In addition, peculiarly uncomfortable feelings of tightness and pressure, like a girdle squeezing the body, are often reported, as is numbness. Any part of the body can be affected, but most commonly it is the limbs, neck and head. Demyelination, which leads to the defective conduction of nerve impulses, causes the brain to be misinformed about what is going on in the periphery of the body. Much of the work of the central nervous system is to shut out distracting sensations in order to concentrate on carrying out everyday tasks. Interference with this results in being bombarded with sensations you don't want and can't control, including pain. Some common types of neurological pain are described below.

Headaches aren't generally much different from normal when you have MS. However, tension headaches can persist for weeks or months prior to the onset of MS, and probably result from physical or emotional stress. They can recur periodically for the same reasons. It is important that doctors check whether a headache has a cause other than stress or demyelination and treat it accordingly.

Lhermitte's paraesthesia is a sudden but brief pain down the back and into the legs and arms that occurs when bending the neck. It can vary from a sharp electric shock type of pain to a sensation of tingling or pins and needles. The only way to cope with it is to avoid bending the neck. Wearing a collar support helps.

Optic neuritis is associated with another unpleasant pain, which affects the eyes. Sharp, like the cut of a knife, it is felt when moving one or both eyes. The eyeballs usually feel tender, and there is often an accompanying headache. It may also be associated with blurred vision, which can last from moments to weeks. It probably results from the stretching of the meninges surrounding the swollen optic nerve. Optic neuritis is a common first symptom of MS. It usually lasts no more than a few days. If severe and longer lasting, the pain of it may be relieved by treatment with steroids, such as methylprednisolone.

Pseudoradicular pain, a continuous sciatica-like pain in one leg, part of the trunk or in an arm, can set in and become very troublesome. This pain varies in intensity and may be experienced with clammy coldness or a burning heat. The MS lesions responsible are probably located in the sensory tracks, or roots, of the spinal cord. It is difficult to treat because some drugs, such as Carbamazepine (Tegretol), that relieve the pain usually have the side effect of weakening the muscles and affecting the way you walk by causing the legs to cross in front of each other in a scissor-like movement.

Spasms, which are uncontrollable contractions in the leg or arm muscles, often cause agonising pain for a short time (see page 154). Although prescription medications are available, some people also (unofficially) use cannabis for pain relief.

Trigeminal neuralgia is thought to result from demyelination of the sensory nerve to the face. It is felt on the side of the head or face, and is often triggered by, for example, cold or being touched. It is a very unpleasant, severe stabbing pain, and depressing if it lasts long. It is usually relieved by taking Carbamazepine (Tegretol). If this doesn't work, alcohol injections into the nerve may be effective.

SECONDARY MS PAIN

Often referred to as musculoskeletal pain because it frequently results from stress and strain on the muscles, ligaments, joints and bones, secondary pain is a by-product of MS. You may feel it in the hips, tailbone, legs and arms, and it generally occurs when you have been immobile for a while, perhaps sitting in a wheelchair for a long time. Lower back pain is particularly common, and is exacerbated by poor posture and strained walking patterns. Pain like this is often controlled by everyday painkillers, such

as paracetamol or ibuprofen. Other secondary pain associated with MS results from pressure sores and infections.

TREATING PAIN

We are all individual, so people with MS will need to
experiment to find out the best method of relieving their
particular pain. Doctors recommend trying conventional
drugs first before turning to less orthodox means of
control, such as biofeedback or acupuncture. Because MS
pain originates directly from the ways in which MS affects
the body, the drugs prescribed will vary. Inevitably it takes
time to find out which type or combination of drugs suits
you best and in which dosage. Remember, it usually takes
time for the effective dose to build up. Don't be surprised
if you find you have been prescribed anti-epileptic or
anti-depressant drugs: both are equally effective in treating nerve pain. Antidepressants, for example, are helpful
because they modify the way the central nervous system
reacts to pain.

Generally speaking, if you suffer from muscle-type
pain, you need to move about more and keep changing
position. If you can't manage an exercise programme, try
spending a few minutes in a rocking chair, or get someone to gently move each limb in turn. Physiotherapy and
massage (gently applied so that the muscles do not go into
spasm) are very beneficial and come highly recommended,
as does yoga. Both physiotherapy and yoga exercises help
create good habits that improve posture and breathing.
Sometimes a physiotherapist or other health professional
will suggest using a transcutaneous nerve stimulation
(TENS) machine to provide pain relief. This passes a weak

electric current over the area of pain. It works brilliantly for many, but not all. (All these treatments are covered in more detail in Chapter 5.)

Occupational therapists are also skilled in helping to lessen pain. One way they do this is by assessing your daily activities and suggesting alternatives to keep pain at bay. They also provide equipment that offers support and ease, such as seating and pressure-relief cushions. They will even check that you are lying on the right sort of mattress, and perhaps suggest trying a water bed or one that can be adjusted. They can also help you experiment with placing pillows for optimum support. If you can cope with the feel of warm water, you may find that your muscles respond by relaxing and are more easily moved. Exercising in water is particularly good for strengthening muscles. Jill literally got back on her feet again after a relapse by exercising regularly in the local swimming pool over a number of months. In fact, she did this after two relapses, and the second time worked even better than the first. Sensation pains often respond to the application of greater pressure, heat or cold.

If all else fails, a doctor will refer you to a specialist pain clinic. As part of the treatment, they will explain the emotional and psychological components of pain. All too quickly pain can become the focus of everything that is wrong in life. It is the strongest statement the body can make as it screams for attention. It gives you a legitimate reason to go to a doctor for help.

LIVING WITH PAIN

Pain affects you in many ways. It stops you being fully involved in life, often forcing you to withdraw from the company of others to suffer in isolation. It is depressing, and can push some people towards thoughts of suicide. When you are putting up with pain, your thinking shuts down and you can't be bothered about life around you or concerned about the problems of others. Your senses are affected – being touched can be so sore, lights painfully bright and glaring, hearing loud, discordant and jumbled, heat exhausting and enervating, cold tooth-grinding and numbing, and damp bone-aching. Pain sets everything on edge.

However, pain also allows you a voice. It gets attention and sympathy from those who see your distress. It allows you to avoid unpleasant situations and to get out of doing what you don't like. It gives you reasons to cover up your feelings or express them in an outburst. It gives you power to get people to do what you want.

Living with pain can persist when the physical reason for the pain has long gone. Pain can become a way of life if you have tolerated it for a long time. That can be countered by finding ways of bringing back enjoyment, fun and laughter into life. Many people remark on the fact that they can forget their pain while they are doing something they enjoy, or spending time with friends they like. Being cheerful and outgoing has a positive effect on the body, producing a kind of chemical reaction that deadens certain pain. There is obviously some truth in the proverb that a merry heart does you as much good as medicine.

Sexual problems

Oliver is a good-looking, virile young man whose MS was affecting his sex life. He needed to reach out, love and be loved in his marriage, but the fact that he could not maintain an erection and suffered occasional impotence had put paid to any lovemaking as far as his wife was concerned. He just could not perform conventionally, and his wife was not prepared to accept any other options sexually. They shut off from each other, stopped trying and stopped communicating their need for each other. He felt guilty because he was unable to satisfy his wife, and they both hurt badly when it seemed that the sexual part of their relationship was over. As a result, Oliver found himself attracted to someone at work, and before long was involved in a secret love affair in which he and his new partner found and enjoyed alternative ways of making love.

Oliver is an example of how a sexual problem can be allowed to go unresolved and cause detrimental separation between partners. It also illustrates the fact that there are always other options when it comes to expressing love. Unlike Oliver, you may never be affected sexually. For instance, when it comes to sexual libido, most people with MS experience a normal drive, a few experiencing an increased one. When MS does interfere with sexual activity, it is inability or reduced ability in the physical expression of sex that is most apparent, although psychological factors are of equal importance. The sexual problems that result differ from person to person, vary between relapse and remission, and are affected by fatigue. The 'too tired tonight' line takes on extra significance with MS.

Men with MS may become impotent, find it difficult to get and maintain an erection, and be aware of changes in the timing, nature and sensation of ejaculation. Women with MS may lack sensation because they lose clitoral engorgement, and may also notice a lack of vaginal lubrication. Spasms in the thigh muscles may occur, making it difficult to have intercourse. For both men and women, it is usually necessary to try out new positions when there is muscular weakness, spasm or rapid fatigue.

FINDING SOLUTIONS

The reasons for sexual problems may be neurological, emotional, or a mixture of the two. It is certainly possible to get help with emotional problems, and it is also possible to find alternative ways of expressing love sexually if the problem is a result of demyelination. Some doctors, counsellors and psychotherapists specialize in helping people with sexual problems. People make love for a host of good reasons, and there is every reason to continue lovemaking even if MS tries to interfere. Sexuality is a vital part of a person's total personality. When you are satisfied sexually, you enjoy a completeness that pervades the whole of you. The reverse is also true. If there are problems and pressures in other parts of your life, your sex life feels the effect.

Even before diagnosis, it is quite likely that MS was already affecting sexual activity. It may have caused fatigue, or unexplained moodiness, or direct loss of sexual function. That will have placed a strain on sexual relationships. Once people know they have MS, they may fear that sexual activity will make their condition worse, though this is in fact highly unlikely unless they allow themselves to become overtired. A little discreet forward planning can normally overcome that problem.

To cope well sexually, you first need to consider your

definition of sexual activity. If you insist on narrowly defining it as the ability to have sexual intercourse conventionally, you are limiting your sexual expression and satisfaction. It is legitimate to discover that there really is no right way, and no need for 'shoulds' in a good, loving sexual relationship. On the other hand, there is plenty of room for discovering new ways of relating.

You also need to become aware of the problems anyone can have in a sexual relationship, and then consider the added problems of MS. Any man with impotence experiences frustration and tends to avoid intercourse because he is afraid of repeated failure. If MS is likely to be the cause and it threatens to be so permanently, then the man's confidence will be knocked twice over. Similarly, a woman may avoid intercourse because she can't enjoy it in the way she used to, and feel that she has failed too, even if there is MS to blame. Both have lost a means of expressing love sexually and spontaneously, a loss that needs to be grieved about before new approaches can be found.

It is also a common experience for those who feel

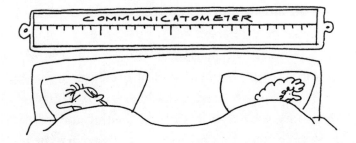

... SEX EASILY BECOMES THE SCAPEGOAT FOR ANY SHAKY MARRIAGE   IT IS A SORT OF BAROMETER, REGISTERING ADVERSELY ANY BREAKDOWN IN COMMUNICATION ...

unattractive, for whatever reason, to believe that they are unlovable and do not warrant sexual relations. If they are also struggling to accept their MS and whatever disability, visible or invisible, that goes with it, they may find that they distance themselves from a sexual partner and ignore or negate the love offered. Or the reverse may be true. They may so crave the reassurance that they are still lovable, that they make unacceptable demands to try and compensate for the negative feelings they have about themselves.

Sex easily becomes the scapegoat for any shaky marriage. It is a sort of barometer, registering adversely any breakdown in communication and closeness. It is sensitive to unexpressed feelings, especially a backlog of anger. If the physical effects of MS on sexual function are not taken into account, there is plenty of scope for misunderstanding. Unresolved sexual problems can become reason enough for your relationship to flounder.

It is easy to fear that a partner will seek sexual satisfaction elsewhere. In the main, such fears are unfounded. Feelings of jealousy may be more strongly felt, partly as a result of the effect MS can have on the emotions. There may be, after all, many more opportunities for a partner to make new relationships, but frequently that partner feels as much jealousy when the person with MS has to be cared for by nursing staff at home or in hospital.

If someone becomes disabled to the degree where he or she needs help with washing, feeding and toileting, and a partner takes this on for them, there may be a change of emphasis in the relationship. There is a potential role conflict when a partner becomes more of a nurse than a lover. Physical contact can easily become limited to the basic essentials of nursing care. There may actually be a need to confront this by specifically encouraging affectionate sexual contact. If it is finally decided to discontinue a sexual relationship, this decision should always be reached mutually and not by default.

There are three basic needs to fulfil if you want a good sexual relationship.

Communicate well. This involves expressing your feelings and being willing to talk frankly and without embarrassment. It helps to share specifically what you like and dislike sexually, what you expect in the relationship, and what approaches to sexual activity you are willing to take.

Preserve intimacy. You deserve to keep a deep and intimate closeness. If one partner has MS, preserving intimacy may involve finding new ways of being close, which at first may feel inadequate, but which are certainly worth investing in. If intercourse is either impossible or ill-advised, caressing, stroking and long, warm hugs help maintain sexual closeness. Most people also find it best to continue to sleep in the same bed. If MS leads to a period in hospital or long-term care away from home, special arrangements may have to be made to keep intimate times going.

Explore and experiment. People with MS may have to make the best of a bad situation, and initially feel too unnatural and frightened to try new approaches. But if they really want to give pleasure as well as to receive it, it is important to seek information on alternative ways of making love, making use of different techniques, sexual aids and more comfortable positions.

It is also important to know how to cope with incontinence problems and catheters, and maintain careful personal hygiene. There are excellent books on the market, some written for the general public and others specifically to cover sex and disability. Several organizations also exist to give advice and help in this area (see page 284). You may also consider seeing a counsellor who specializes in helping couples with sexual problems.

Incontinence

For a symptom that can often be successfully managed, if not completely eradicated, incontinence is a problem that assumes mega proportions. Elaine, a nurse, dreaded it more than any other symptom, a fear stemming back to her own toilet-training as a child. It became such a bogey in her mind that she worked herself into a state of gloomy depression and introversion. What she needed was reassurance that if she ever did experience incontinence problems, she could rely on a wealth of expertise to help her cope.

The fact that many people are embarrassed by bodily functions, such as going to the toilet, cannot be dismissed. It is one of those natural activities people easily learn to be unnatural about. It helps not to be prudish. People have no problem accepting that babies are incontinent, but often fuss and fret when emotional problems, accidents, disease or old age result in an incontinence problem in someone past babyhood. Incontinence is a very widespread problem, especially for women, but in genteel society it is a topic one would rather not mention. Even among women with MS, around 20 per cent can blame their incontinence on something other than the disease. Those who suffer from it, for whatever reason, do continue to lead normal active lives once they have received treatment or are given adequate methods of coping with it.

BLADDER INCONTINENCE

The most common form of incontinence is a loss of bladder control, which means that you pass urine when you don't plan to. When young children are toilet-trained, they learn bladder control by programming their brains to interrupt the natural reflex action of passing water without restraint. What they learn to control consciously are the sphincter muscle at the neck of the bladder and the detrusor muscles in the bladder wall. They learn to 'hold on' and pass water only when appropriate. If the nerve pathways in the spinal cord transmitting messages between the brain and the bladder muscles are damaged by demyelination, this directly affects the 'warning system'. One common effect of this is feeling the need to dash to the toilet again and again. It makes for a very tiresome lifestyle, forcing you never to stray far from a toilet. It is often worth warning friends and colleagues about it in a brief, factual but light-hearted way. This is the type of incontinence doctors refer to when they ask if you have any problems with frequency and urgency. Normally the detrusor muscles and sphincter cooperate in either storing or emptying the bladder – one of them is always 'on the go', either relaxing or contracting. *Urge incontinence* is when the bladder empties almost as soon as the desire to pass urine is felt. The detrusor muscles in the bladder wall become overactive, go into a spasm without warning, and the bladder has to act. It just can't wait for you to give the go-ahead. *Reflex incontinence* is similar in result, only this time the message from the brain doesn't get through to the sphincter to check the reflex emptying of the bladder. This is also what happens with bed-wetting.

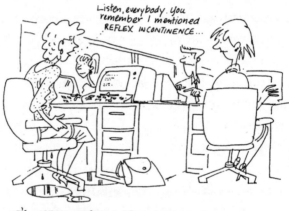

IT'S OFTEN WORTH WARNING YOUR FRIENDS AND COLLEAGUES ABOUT INCONTINENCE IN A BRIEF, FACTUAL AND LIGHT-HEARTED WAY ..

Occasionally, people with MS suffer the reverse problem – *retention* – when you want to empty your bladder but can't. It is prevented by a spasm or strong contraction of the sphincter, or because the normal coordination between the sphincter and detrusor muscles goes awry. Sometimes urine is retained because the sphincter doesn't open properly, but is then suddenly squeezed out because there are detrusor spasms in the bladder wall. This affects the flow, which is usually slow and interrupted, and leads to incomplete emptying. Unfortunately, people with MS can't always feel if the bladder is completely empty, and any urine left behind can aggravate incontinence.

No wonder some people carry a 'I can't wait because I've got MS' card to flash in crowded toilets, available in four languages from the MS Society. In terms of self-help, there is value in regularly practising pelvic floor exercises. Professional help begins with an assessment of the bladder's ability to empty, using a specific urine flow test, administered by a nurse or continence adviser. A flow of over 100 ml is generally controlled by intermittent self-catheterization, which is when you insert a catheter to empty the bladder fully. A lesser flow is normally treated with drugs to reduce bladder contractions. Many people find that learning to self-catheterize is a relief in more ways than one. By being able to choose when to empty the bladder, they gain the control needed to cope with outings and social activities.

A word of warning about not taking in enough fluid. Sometimes people with incontinence problems mistakenly cut down their fluid intake. This can have very serious consequences because the urine becomes more concentrated, which may irritate the bladder and increase the risk of urinary tract infections (UTIs). UTIs are painful, very weakening and potentially dangerous, whether caused by infection or from the effect of MS on the muscles of the bladder, and require early drug intervention.

In severe MS there is often a connection between bladder problems and walking difficulties. If MS progresses and mobility becomes more laboured, incontinence is likely to become a bigger issue. Protective measures, such as special pads, underwear and bedding, need to be taken.

One practical way of coping with incontinence is to use some sort of indwelling catheter. An added advantage of using a catheter is that it helps to ward off bladder infections, which can easily develop if any urine is left unpassed in the bladder. A catheter, left in place with a bag or valve attached, is very practical if you are generally confined to a wheelchair or bed. Most catheters are fitted in the urethra by a nurse. Sometimes a urologist fits a supra-pubic catheter under local or general anaesthetic into the abdomen via a small incision. This is a more appropriate catheter if you have leg spasms (and it makes for easier sexual activity) Both urethral and supra-pubic catheters need changing at least every 12 weeks. Occasionally, surgical interventions are offered. If you self-catheterize, an ileocystoplasty helps increase the bladder's capacity and also reduces spasms. A urostomy diverts urine into a bag attached to the skin.

BOWEL INCONTINENCE

Most of us find the bowels difficult to talk about. It's hard to find the right words, and most people feel embarrassed, if not ashamed. The two main problems that may develop are constipation and bowel incontinence. You can have constipation without having incontinence, or suffer from both. Constipation is much commoner than bowel incontinence.

In contrast to all that is known about the effect of multiple sclerosis on the bladder, much less is known about how MS affects the bowel. What is clear is that the disease can be responsible for a sluggish gut, for muscles that sometimes refuse to coordinate and push, relax or hold on, or for a loss of sensation so that you don't realize that you really need to 'go'.

Constipation can often be helped by choosing a wholefood diet rich in bran, wholemeal bread and pasta, brown rice and fresh fruit and vegetables, which provide the roughage needed to guard against constipation. It's also important to drink enough fluid and avoid too much refined food. If dietary changes do not do the trick, seek medical advice on which suppositories or laxatives to use. Getting into a regular and comfortable routine that gives you privacy and enough time to relax is important, especially if you rely on carers who come into your home. Constipation is more common among people who live a sedentary life. If you have mobility problems, you may need to compensate by doing exercises of some sort to benefit not only the bowels but also your health in general. Certain drugs can cause constipation, so check with your doctor to see if there are alternatives.

Loss of control of both the bladder and bowel is called double incontinence.

Incontinence can become a severe problem during a relapse. Normal or much improved control will return spontaneously during remission. Incontinence may always be an MS symptom, or one that becomes more of a problem if the disease becomes progressive. It may also increase with age, which is true for the aging population in general. The person to go to for help initially is your GP or MS nurse, who may refer you to a specialist or nurse continence adviser. Alternatively, you can always self-refer to most NHS Continence Advisory Services. MS and continence organizations (see pages 284 and 291) all offer invaluable information on coping with incontinence, plus detailed advice on drugs, catheterization, pads and various appliances that are widely available. With this expert help, most people will be able to cope. Whether incontinence is temporary or permanent, it is always worthwhile getting the right advice.

Cognitive difficulties

Although you may never experience any cognitive problems (difficulties with memory and concentration), around 50 per cent of people with MS report doing so, at least to a mild degree. These difficulties can happen at any time, without any connection to other MS symptoms, the type of MS you have, how long you've had it, the severity of the disease, or whether you show any signs of physical disability or not. Naturally it will help if you can laugh it off as just a nuisance that gets worse when you are overtired. However, it can be a matter of real concern if it interferes with everyday living. Finding coping strategies to minimize cognitive impairment makes life easier and boosts morale.

Certain specific cognitive problems are typical of MS. One of the most common is to do with short-term memory – being unable to recall recent events spontaneously, especially in any detail. It feels as if you are being faced with a closed door, which only swings wide open when the right trigger or prompt acts to let you rediscover in all clarity what you couldn't access before. Sometimes it helps to ease off even trying to remember. Idle in neutral and sometimes that 'door' opens without effort. Another common but related cognitive effect of

MS is not remembering to do something you had intended to. When you find you keep forgetting, it's hard not to get cross with yourself and become fearful. Understandably, it's easy to fear the worst and lose confidence, but there are strategies for coping with both these difficulties. MS does not have the same negative effects on recognition memory as it does on recall or remembering, so you can retrieve information you have previously stored away by being 'tipped off', so to speak. When it begins to take so much more time and effort to bring to mind something that happened or remember what you still need to do, it makes sense to start jotting things down, keeping a diary, making lists or even using an alarm clock or bleeper so that you have information and reminders at hand. Quite a few people find that these cognitive problems increase before a relapse, or occur at the tail end of one, as you are beginning to recover again.

Concentration can also be noticeably affected. Perhaps the practicalities of having MS shift your mind elsewhere. For example, it's vital to know where the nearest loo is, or how best to negotiate transferring from one place to another. Certainly people with MS find that attention and concentration tend to waver, especially if they are interrupted or try to do more than one thing at a time. Getting things done often seems to take longer and require greater effort. That, in turn, can have negative effects on work and relationships. Sometimes you can work for only short periods of time and may actively need to shut out any distractions. It's important to check you've understood all that's involved – not only facts, but how other people fit in too. You may also need to ensure you are making yourself clear. (Preparing yourself beforehand is sound practice.) Fatigue seems to play a significant part here. It's wise to build in breaks to recuperate and allow yourself to assimilate what's been happening. Also, if those around you know how fatigued you are, they will readily make allowances and accept a different approach or the need for more time.

Similarly, problem solving, and even finding the right word or train of thought quickly enough to join in a discussion, can become problematic. It's not always easy to know where to start working through a problem and how to achieve a goal step by step. Sometimes people find they get stuck in some sort of 'tunnel vision', unable to see the bigger picture. Once you recognize that is happening, you may have to diplomatically bring a premature close to any further discussion or negotiation until you are in the right frame of mind or mood to consider other options. Again, fatigue appears to aggravate difficulties with problem solving.

Cognitive difficulties are also temporarily worsened if you are suffering from pain, depression or a relapse. And once you get stressed and confused, things seem to get even worse. One way of coping is to withdraw from the fray for a while. Another valuable skill is to foster an atmosphere of goodwill so that you can tell others when you are fatigued, need time to think or try a different approach.

Similarly, if you get trapped in a nondescript sort of life lacking the stimulation you used to get from work, hobbies or socializing, this is also likely to have a negative effect. It is often suggested that since a majority of people with MS are pretty bright go-getters, used to being spot-on, they are overcritical of even average memory loss. Nevertheless, any cognitive impairment is accompanied by a certain amount of uncertainty and fear, so it is important to check out what is going on with your GP, who can arrange for a professional neuro-psychological assessment.

Depression

People with MS frequently suffer depression. It's unclear just how much this is to do with the challenges and reactions to being diagnosed with the disease. About one quarter of newly diagnosed people aged 18–45 experience a major depressive episode. It is also a fact that people with MS are almost three times as likely to suffer from major depression at some time compared with the general population. Research studies into how much depression is clinically part and parcel of MS itself are as yet inconclusive, and there is no evidence of a link between depression and levels of disability or the length of time you have had MS. One complicating factor is that MS and depression share symptoms in common, such as fatigue. However, even in contrast to people with other neurological conditions, people with MS do have a greater incidence of depression – the sort of depression that is often distinguished by greater irritation and frustration.

It is understandable that the shock and implications of an MS diagnosis might set off a train of reactive depression. It propels you into an uncertain future, where your previous assumptions about your lifestyle, employment, earnings and relationships no longer hold true. It's worth noting that after diagnosis your partner is just as likely to be depressed as you are. Learning about what may lie ahead can indeed unsettle and alarm. Anyone who isn't a bit depressed and scared at hearing the possibility of developing disability or loss of independent living would be abnormal. So some of the depression around MS is clearly a normal protective reaction to the new situation you are facing.

Neurologists with a particular interest in helping people with MS to cope better will support their patients in finding ways to treat depression. This may include treatment with drugs, or encouragement to try some form of psychological support, such as cognitive behaviour therapy. Some people with MS prefer 'natural' remedies and find they do the trick. Without doubt, success in treating depression is indeed a load lifted, and invariably enables the individual to cope better with MS.

Speech difficulties

It may be true that communication between people relies as much upon body language as the words we say, but we all rely heavily on being able to speak and on having our words understood. Speech is a highly complex process, which depends on finely controlled and coordinated muscles. Any adverse physical effect on the muscles involved inevitably impairs our ability to speak. Sadly, MS can occasionally produce such effects. These are very individual, varying from scarcely perceptible to more severe, and they can also vary from day to day or even hour to hour. Certainly fatigue worsens any speech problems. Some people with MS say that on low-energy days they notice that their speech slows down and sounds softer, and sometimes their words are slightly slurred.

Reactions to speech impairment are very individual. The slightest difficulty proves devastating for some people, while others with greater problems take it in their stride and stay buoyant, confidently exploring any means possible to keep in touch. There is no doubt that familiarity helps: it is easier to communicate fully with people you are relaxed with and who enjoy finding ways of ensuring they understand you. Carers of people with severe speech problems become resourceful in finding alternative ways of communicating. Similarly, Graham's ability to chat up his nurses made many an unsuspecting one blush! He certainly managed to find ways to express his thoughts and wishes much of the time, but he also experienced the frustration of not being able to communicate in detail. Not being understood feels like being excluded or dismissed, and is distressing for both parties. Maintaining a good relationship that thrives on kindness and respect is therefore vital.

It is wise to consult a speech and language therapist early on for tips on how to cope. Your GP, neurologist or any health professional will put you in touch with someone suitably qualified. Speech therapists expect to work differently with each individual. They know that success in exploring how to keep channels of communication open depends on building good rapport and trust with their clients and families. They know ways to ensure that breathing is improved and will introduce exercises that may be helpful at certain times. In the most serious cases of speech impediment, communication aid equipment may be recommended. The suppliers of this are extremely skilled in teaching how to use it, and normally work together with the speech therapists.

Psychological struggles

The greatest psychological struggles people with MS have to face are to do with fear and prejudice – from themselves as well as others. This confrontation first occurs at diagnosis, then on and off afterwards, if or when the symptoms of MS prove disabling in any way. To be aware of this situation helps. To be able to give it a name and recognize it for what it is limits its power. A person can then choose what weight to give it in his or her life.

FEAR

Even if MS remains invisible, those who have it will never be entirely free of occasional niggling fears. They are those momentary 'what if' fears that should be acknowledged, but then dismissed. Chances are that if ever these fears do become reality, you will find the strength to cope somehow. That is also true for fears more firmly based on fact. Accept that they may be valid at some future point, but that for now they can be put aside.

There are times when fears can build into a panic. Many factors can be involved in this – personality type, experience of life, relationships, the situation at home, work, general state of health and, not least, the fact of living with a neurological disease affecting the central nervous system. Such panic is invariably temporary – it will pass. There is no need to do anything about it except to allow time for it to release and settle. People who habitually experience panic attacks may choose to get professional support in overcoming them.

PREJUDICE

There is a very real but unspoken prejudice against disability and whatever indicates the presence of disability. It may be a prejudice you are already aware of in yourself or others. It can even be a prejudice that people with MS feel towards themselves. While it is more common to experience this prejudice in the face of visible disablement, it is also possible to experience it when facing the effects of invisible symptoms.

The prejudice against disability is obvious in people who grumble about those in wheelchairs cluttering up the pavement or shops, and who are impatient to get past someone walking slowly with a stick. What is happening to people with the prejudice is that the aids – wheelchair or stick – get in the way and obscure the personality of the individual using them. The observers focus on what frightens and threatens them and are unable to take a broader view. The more severe the disability, the greater the threat.

MS, with its fluctuating pattern and periods of deterioration during relapse, poses a threat. Those who have to confront MS are placed in a quandary as they consider how severe their disability is, what its long-term effect could possibly be, and how predictable and controllable its outcome. The conclusions drawn may determine whether or not help is offered and acceptance given. If neither is readily on offer, the person with MS will feel rejected and isolated.

It is a fact that certain illnesses carry more of a stigma than others. For example, heart attacks do not appear to have the stigma that MS does. The causes, treatments and prevention of heart attacks are understood and clear-cut in a way that MS is not. Frequently people with MS, their families and friends may unconsciously react in ways that imply they are somehow ashamed of the disease and its symptoms. The mystery of what causes it and the unpredictability of its course make them defensive. This defensiveness is put down to MS, but is more to do with the stigma of the disease. MS has a bad press: it is feared and threatening. The stigma of it is something else to grapple with and resolve, but you should never take on the responsibility for the effect of MS upon others. You may be able to make them better aware of it, and you may also have to learn to accept that you can do nothing to change other people's reactions. Some people will avoid contact with anyone with MS and feel guilty about it. They are struggling with their own inability to overcome prejudice against a disabling illness. Indeed, it can be more disabling for them to cope with the stigma than for the person with MS to cope with the disease. They find themselves watching carefully to make sure they say the 'right' things and not let it be obvious that they are finding the situation difficult. They emphasize the positive at all times because they are afraid to feel and express any negative emotions, especially anger, towards someone with MS, in case the prejudice slips out and is revealed. It must be stressed that this is rarely a prejudice that anyone admits to. It seldom surfaces at a conscious level. It is not calculated in any way. It is an unconscious fear, with far-reaching effects on relationships.

This section has focused on the way that MS can limit and change social relationships. People with MS need to be aware that the disease can disable not only them, but also their families, friends and others they come across, albeit in a different way. The family in particular runs the risk of being most seriously affected by prejudice against disability, and may also experience the effects of stigmatization. It happens most easily when MS is handled as something fragile that they are afraid to talk about normally and dare not laugh at. They get into a pattern of allowing MS too important a place in their lives. It is people themselves who count; the practicalities of coping with disability should not intrude or predominate. Sadly, however, MS at its worst does demand a high degree of physical care and attention, inevitably placing a heavy burden on those who do the caring. If this happens, support of a special kind is needed to minimize the intrusion of MS so that it is still possible to maintain warmth and openness in relationships.

When caring becomes a crisis

There will be times when there is a need to reflect on the meaning of life and death in the light of one's own vulnerability. It is normal and healthy to do so, and having MS is a good enough reason to take stock. Some prefer to ponder on their own, while others want to work out ideas with the help of others. Often it is easier to do so with someone understanding, who has a distance from your immediate family and closest friends. It will help you to voice what is going on inside you, and give you courage to consider the changes that you would like to initiate in order to meet the future. At some stage it is wise to involve those close to you in discussing your future, provided you and they can cope with it.

PLAN AHEAD

No one knows what lies ahead, but it makes good sense to begin to build into relationships what is needed to survive any eventuality. In practical terms this might mean arranging that people with MS and those caring for them can have time apart.

People need a break and space for themselves. Although this is especially important if the person with MS becomes severely disabled, it also holds true for their carers. When people are together for 24 hours a day, 365 days of the year, there is a very real danger of their relationship becoming claustrophobic and stifling. One way of avoiding this is for people with MS to learn early on how to accept physical care and attention from others, and still retain control, dignity and a sense of humour. It is very important, if possible, to make sure that one person, particularly your partner, does not have sole responsibility for washing, feeding or toileting.

FIND HELP

District nurses or home carers are usually available to come in and take responsibility for routine nursing and physical care for severe MS or very acute relapses. Suitable nursing staff may be paid for under the conditions of some private medical insurance schemes. There is also the Crossroads Care attendance scheme, a network of carers throughout the country, who contract to come in and relieve on a regular basis. Using such outside help allows some space between people who need to be cared for and their family or friends who normally do the caring.

ADMIT THE STRAIN

It is unrealistic to expect any single relationship to supply everything you want at any time and on demand, even if you are related by blood or marriage. Yvonne went back home to live when she needed some looking after. However, she had never had an easy relationship with her mother, and although they both tried hard, in the end they had to admit that Yvonne would be better off in a hostel catering for the disabled, where she could still welcome occasional visits. An alternative form of support, which may enable someone to remain independent for longer, is to have a skilled assistance or companion dog, which is taught specific skills to meet the daily living needs of its owner.

There is no denying the strain involved in living day in and day out with disability, especially when you are largely physically dependent on others. It's all too easy to become confined to four walls, and find yourself and those caring for you becoming isolated from the mainstream of life. There is distress whenever you grapple with a slow slide towards any sort of incapacity, relief at any halting, and joy when, despite all indications to the contrary, remission takes place.

Carers in such situations, especially any whose partner has developed primary progressive MS while still young, often face losing the cut and thrust that characterizes an equal relationship. Even though love still binds them together, there is nonetheless a sad, deep sense of loss if the person with MS becomes seriously disabled. Fast deterioration is fraught with change and challenge. It feels as if you have to gallop to keep abreast of the unpredictability. If severe disability becomes chronic, people often report that the person with MS seems distanced, self-absorbed rather than participating. Inevitably this impacts on all family relationships.

Dealing with the practicalities of being cared for can eat up so many hours and so much energy that it is difficult to hold on to some of the trimmings so that life has quality and is not just a matter of existence. Twice a week Olga, despite severe disability, went back to her old school where she had been a teacher. There she spent a couple of hours listening and helping the children to read. They loved the attention, found her wheelchair a novelty, and never minded that she could not move her arms and legs or talked in a funny way. She knew she was fulfilling a useful function.

RESPITE CARE

The routine of caring and being cared for takes a toll on everyone involved, so it is helpful to have a short break and spend some time away from each other. The name for this is respite care. Short-term breaks for people with MS are often available at home or at a day centre, or might involve a stay in a care home, hospice or other facility. Many people find it helps to plan respite care into their year, as an opportunity for rehabilitation. Certainly, if you choose a respite care centre that specializes in supporting people with MS, there will be the added bonus of input from a wide range of professionals with expertise in the challenges of MS. They could offer, for example, help with particular health problems, such as cognitive impairment, or different types of rehabilitation therapy. Some centres offer physiotherapy and complementary treatments such as aromatherapy, reflexology or occasionally hydrotherapy, which are very beneficial in terms of relaxation and well-being. Emergency care is sometimes also possible.

Finding the right sort of break for you takes a bit of planning, for you need to maximize the benefits as well as ensuring you get value for money.

The MS Society keeps an up-to-date *Respite Care Directory*, which contains a list of potential care providers, some of whom have been awarded the status of 'Preferred Provider' to signify that they have met certain essential criteria to provide care for people with MS, especially those with advanced and complex needs. In addition, the MS Society operates four care homes of its own. Other charities, such as the Leonard Cheshire Foundation, the John Grooms Housing Association and Vitalise (see pages 294 and 299), also provide quality care.

Respite care is expensive because of the high costs of staffing, especially for high-dependency care. However, financial assistance is often available from statutory agencies, such as social services and health authorities, and also from a number of trusts, charities and the like. The local branch of the MS Society may also be able to assist in funding respite care.

LONG-TERM RESIDENTIAL CARE

There may come a time when long-term residential care needs to be considered. This can often be an emotionally charged decision to make, and for many people it seems like an admission of failure. It is not easy for a partner or family to have to admit, for whatever reason, that they cannot manage to continue caring for someone at home. Residential care in a private, local authority, health authority or voluntary-run home is an option that makes good sense when someone needs constant personal nursing care. It is certainly an option that should be considered when the possibilities of additional help from district nurses or care assistants coming in on a daily basis have been exhausted. Remember, though, that while people with MS may understand that they need special nursing care that perhaps only a residential home can give, they will often be reluctant to move from an intimate, family-type situation to being part of a larger, less personal group. They will fear isolation and wonder whether their family and friends will actually remember to come and visit them after a while.

While it is true that some families squeeze out a member with MS and jump at the chance of residential care, the reverse can also happen. Relationships previously under strain because of all the sheer hard physical work and long hours can and do improve dramatically. Some individuals with MS prefer residential care because it gets them the care they need and leaves them with more energy for visitors. Visits become a pleasure, and people enjoy a renewed and relaxed warmth with each other. Veronica found her MS easier to cope with after getting out of a disastrous marriage and moving to an excellent care home. The fact that a circle of caring friends and family paid her regular visits and took her out improved her quality of life.

PALLIATIVE CARE

When the quality of life is seriously compromised or threatened, little can be done beyond offering comfort or pain relief. This is called palliative care, and is offered by professionals to both the patient and those close to them. A condition such as MS, with its acute episodes or progressive disability, may sometimes demand palliative care expertise. This might focus on managing symptoms, or offer opportunities to explore psychological, social or spiritual issues that may come to the fore with severe MS, and find resolution and peace of mind. Palliative care may be appropriate early on after diagnosis, during a severe relapse, or whenever disabling symptoms threaten to get the better of you. It may also be just the right sort of care at the end of life.

Death

One of the taboo subjects in our society is death. Few of us talk about it, yet it is the only certainty after birth. It is best faced with calmness and dignity, as part of what T.S. Eliot called a 'magnificent pattern'. If you have MS, you cannot help but die with it or of it. Your MS may have nothing at all to do with your dying or it may be a contributory or primary factor. Whichever is the case, it is wise to ensure that all personal affairs are in order and that, as far as possible, you are at peace with yourself and with others.

One way of approaching death is to anticipate the best and worst scenarios, and to consider how you can do something positive about them. Should ill health prove overwhelming, it is normal to feel depressed, without control and hope, so some individuals choose to make clear in advance their wishes regarding how they want to be treated should their condition deteriorate. Melinda was adamant that she didn't want to end up as a 'blob', so she decided to find out about making a 'living will' (also called an 'advance directive'). Someone from her local palliative care team spent time talking it through with Melinda and her husband. The understanding support they received almost made them give up the idea because they felt that if similar care and concern were guaranteed at the end of life, they could ask for no better. But, just in case, Melinda still went ahead, and with the help of her solicitor drew up a legal document stating her personal wishes not to receive artificial nutrition, hydration or life-prolonging medication should she ever reach the state when these might be applied. A pre-prepared form available from the Terrence Higgins Trust, appropriately witnessed, will also be respected as a legally binding document.

Many people with MS have a real interest in research, keep up to date with the latest trends, and eagerly volunteer to participate in drug trials. They are very keen to help researchers find a cause and cure for MS. Robert felt that the most personal gift he could make to the MS community would be to donate his tissue directly to research. He and his family were both pleased and proud about their decision to make this bequest to the UK MS Tissue Bank (see pages 258 and 287). Like all the other donors, some with MS and others without (for both types of tissue are essential), they believe that Robert's contribution will be vital to MS research.

FIVE

Help for those with MS

Anyone with a chronic disease such as MS is bound to be bombarded with concern and contradictory advice. Some of the treatments and sources of help outlined here may work to your advantage, but none is likely to be responsible for a cure because it would be difficult to provide objective proof of one. The capricious nature of MS means that sometimes people begin to improve regardless of treatment. It is worth bearing in mind that some 20 per cent of people with MS do well without any

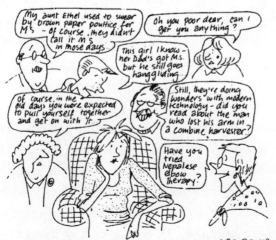

WITH A CHRONIC DISEASE LIKE MS YOU ARE BOUND
TO BE BOMBARDED WITH CONCERN AND CONTRADICTORY ADVICE.

interventions, while another 20 per cent will not do well whatever intervention is tried.

MS is managed in a host of different ways, but basically there are two therapeutic approaches:

- Drugs or treatments that actually modify the disease
- Therapies that ease or reduce specific symptoms (symptomatic treatments)

Both approaches are essential for people with MS, and many of the treatments within them are outlined in this chapter. Alongside the information about conventional, complementary and alternative therapies are tips for healthful living, advice about nutrition and exercise, and even tips about finances. Also outlined is a range of personal support available to people with MS and those closest to them. MS often acts as a catalyst in our lives, so it helps to separate out the different 'threads'. In the best-case scenario this will also include exploring, unravelling and hopefully resolving the emotional and psychological impact of MS on everyone affected by it. The aim is to live healthily and holistically, with body, mind and spirit in harmony.

In the United Kingdom the National Institute for Clinical Excellence (NICE) has addressed the management of multiple sclerosis in the community and in hospitals through its publication *NICE Guidelines for the Treatment and Management of MS* (see page 296). It rightly points to the necessity of providing good evidence to back up any claims for treatments, including complementary and alternative medicine. In order to do justice to what follows, it is important to get a handle on how drugs in particular are developed to either modify the course of MS or treat its symptoms. Ultimately you must choose your own pathway through everything that is on offer.

Drug development and clinical trials

Whenever a new treatment is publicized it is greeted with hope and excitement, but it is important to know how its effects can be evaluated in order to show that it really does work. We hear about many examples of false hope being raised by incorrect reporting in the media, or the release of information before the final and complete results of research are known. It should be remembered that clinical trials of new drugs are also part of the research process. In this case it uses people, rather than animals or cells in dishes, for testing the effects of drugs. Of course, this can only be done after the drugs have been tested using other methods to make sure that they are not dangerous and that they have the potential to change the course of MS in some way. Researchers are aware that animal models of MS are not MS itself, but they can be designed to reproduce the same damage that occurs with MS via the same mechanisms (where they are known). No matter how desperate the need to find new drugs, it is vitally important to test them rigorously before unleashing them on the human body.

One of the greatest problems encountered when evaluating new treatments for MS is the inherent variability of the disease. This means that a treatment that works in one person will not necessarily work in another. This is a problem in all therapeutics, but it is a much bigger problem in MS, and clinical trials must be designed to reflect this. The inherent variability is incorporated either by testing very large numbers of patients, or by restricting the trial to sub-types of MS, or to people at certain stages of MS. Although this can be a source of much frustration to people with MS wishing to take part in clinical trials, it is done in order to improve the chances of actually detecting a significant improvement in symptoms or in the course of MS. If there is too much variability, or 'noise', as it is called, then it is very difficult to see the underlying trends.

The first trials of a new drug in people will be so-called 'safety trials' (what the drug industry calls *phase one trials*). These are carried out in only a small number of people to check for any unexpected side effects that were not predicted by previous testing methods. If the new drugs are considered safe enough, that is free from serious side effects, they will pass on to the next stage of testing, the *phase two trial*. This will involve more people, usually up to 200, and will be carried out over a period of up to a year in most cases. At this second stage it is necessary to consider whether any clinical improvement in your MS is a result of the new therapy or would have happened anyway in the natural course of the disease. This means that the drug trial will be designed so that you and the person evaluating the effect of the new drug (usually a neurologist) will not know whether you are taking the new drug or a dummy drug called a placebo. The power of the human mind is such that just the idea of being given hope through a new drug can change the way we feel and can even improve the symptoms to some degree. For this reason these trials are also called *randomized, double-blind, placebo-controlled trials.* The number of times specific side effects are seen will also be evaluated at this stage.

If the results of phase two trials show that the new therapy has a beneficial effect, which could be an improvement in individual symptoms, a reduction in the number of relapses, a reduction in the accumulation of disability, or improvement in some other aspect of MS that the trial has been designed to test, it will move on to the final stage of testing, the *phase three trial.* The new therapy is now tested on a larger number of people (1,000–2,000) over a longer period, usually up to two or three years. Phase three trials are often carried out internationally so that sufficient people with MS can be recruited to take part, and because physicians can only evaluate so many people on the drug treatments in the time available.

A success in phase three trials means that a pharmaceutical company can then approach the government for a licence to sell the drug as a treatment for MS, a process that we know is not always guaranteed to be successful. The company must prove that the new drug is better than anything currently on sale for MS. You may well ask why so many layers of trials are necessary before a drug can be used for MS. Is it not obvious when something improves the symptoms or course of the disease, and is it not unethical to prevent it being made available? In the end, any therapy will stand or fall according to how beneficial it is to how many people, and taking into account the risk to the taker and the cost in terms of money, time and effort. It is not possible for even very large pharmaceutical companies to absorb the expense of many failed phase three drug trials, each of which costs many millions of pounds. The companies also cannot afford the legal costs if a drug released on to the market is later shown to have serious side effects. The reality is that companies must make a profit from selling new drugs or they will not be able to invest money in developing the next ones. Although the systems put in place by the government and pharmaceutical companies for the development and testing of new therapies may seem imperfect, they are in the main designed to provide the maximum benefit to patients and to protect them.

The number of clinical trials for new treatments for MS has been increasing rapidly in recent years, largely thanks to the large investment in MS research over the past decade. At the time of writing this book (2005), there are about 150 clinical trials going on around the world to test new treatments. This represents a significant investment in terms of both research and drug development. We present here information on some of the drugs currently available that have been shown to alter the course of MS (*disease-modifying drugs*) and a few new ones that are likely to become available in the relatively near future.

Disease-modifying drug therapy

DMDs, as disease-modifying drugs are known, are now widely available for everyone with MS who meets the prescribing criteria. These drugs attempt to change the actual course of MS, slowing it down or even stopping it. They modify the disease in several ways:

- They reduce the number of relapses.
- The relapses are less severe and last less time.
- They decrease the number of lesions visible on MRI scans.

All of this is very positive, but DMDs don't add up to a cure. It is still uncertain whether they will slow down the rate of disability or even stop people becoming disabled. Nor can DMDs reverse any previous permanent damage resulting from MS. But any therapy that minimizes the damage caused by bad MS relapses offers hope, which is why, provided they meet the eligibility criteria, people with MS are given a choice of whether or not to try a disease-modifying drug therapy. These are the first drugs to become available that can really improve the quality of life for a large number of people with MS, although it must be made clear that not everyone experiences benefit.

What disease-modifying drugs are available?

There are two different types of DMDs for MS, four of which are currently licensed for use in the UK. A licensed drug is regarded as both effective and safe to the extent claimed by the manufacturers, who have permission to market it in the UK.

BETA-INTERFERON

Interferons are proteins naturally present in the body, where their function is to help fight viral infections. This means they are vitally important in keeping the immune system functioning well. But only beta-interferon is helpful in MS. The other types, alpha and gamma, are either unhelpful or harmful.

Beta-interferon comes in two types, 1a and 1b. Both do exactly the same job, but are manufactured differently. They reduce MS inflammation and also appear to modify the body's auto-immune reaction responsible for demyelination, at least in the short term.

There are three brands of beta-interferon: Avonex (beta-interferon 1a), Betaferon (beta-interferon 1b) and Rebif (beta-interferon 1a). All three are suitable for long-term use in relapsing and remitting MS, and Betaferon and Rebif are used for some forms of secondary progressive MS.

GLATIRAMER ACETATE

Sold under the brand name Copaxone, this is a completely different drug from beta-interferon. It is composed of protein molecules (amino acids) designed in the laboratory to mimic the structure of one of the main proteins that move up the myelin sheath. In principle, it is thought to act by trying to persuade the immune system to become tolerant to myelin proteins that it recognizes as foreign, thereby stimulating the repair arm of the inflammatory response. It is also used for relapsing and remitting MS.

How DMDs are administered

All the drugs currently available are injected using an automatic injector or autojet, but each in a different way.

Avonex is injected into muscle once a week, while the other three are injected under the skin: Rebif three times a week, Betaferon every other day, and Copaxone daily. Some of these drugs need to be kept cool.

There are certain practical concerns about managing the injections. For instance, Avonex, Rebif and Copaxone come pre-mixed, but Betaferon needs mixing before injecting. Will you find that easy to do, and also will you be able to inject yourself? If not, who can you turn to for help? In addition, you will need cupboard space to store the drug, syringes, needles and special (sharps) box for discarded needles, and fridge space to store medication at the right temperature.

Who qualifies for DMDs?

If you want to consider using a disease-modifying drug, you must first ensure you meet the eligibility criteria set out by the Association of British Neurologists. Your neurologist or MS nurse will be ready to help you. Alternatively, you can look for guidance and the latest eligibility checklist in the literature or on the websites of any of the main MS charities. The most detailed information on DMDs is found on a special independent website (www.msdecisions. org.uk), which also features audio interviews with people with MS, and video clips of how to inject.

Here, in brief, are the criteria for those with relapsing-remitting MS. You must:

• Be able to walk 100 metres without help from another person, but using a stick.

- Have had two clinically definite relapses in the previous two years.
- Be over 18 years old.
- Have no contraindications or reasons why you shouldn't be able to take the drug, e.g. pregnancy or breast-feeding.

If you have secondary progressive MS and want DMD therapy, you must:

- Be able to walk 10 metres without help from anyone, but with a stick.
- Have had two clinically definite relapses in the previous two years confirmed by a neurologist.
- Be over 18 years old.
- Have no contraindications.
- Have experienced only a very minimal increase in disability due to slow progression over the last two years.

As yet there are no disease-modifying drugs for primary progressive MS. The beta-interferons do not appear to have any effect on this type of MS, which suggests that the disease mechanisms involved in primary progressive MS are similar to those occurring during the later stages of non-relapsing secondary progressive MS.

In practice, your neurologist will have the final say over whether you meet the eligibility criteria as he or she knows you and your sort of MS.

It is important to understand that there are also criteria for stopping the use of DMDs. If you plan to have a baby, you should stop DMD therapy at least three months before trying to conceive. If you have relapsing-remitting MS and experience either two disabling relapses, as defined by an examining neurologist, within a 12-month period, or one relapse causing increased disability that lasts for over six months, or move into a phase of not being able to walk with or without assistance for six months, you must also discontinue DMD therapy. With secondary progressive MS, an observable increase in disability over six months is also reason to stop.

DMDs are expensive, but are prescribed under the 'Risk-sharing Scheme', so called because the NHS and the drug companies that produce them are sharing the financial risk of prescribing them – a sort of long-term 'payment by result'.

Choosing which drug to take

There is no best drug – all DMDs are good, and much the same in terms of decreasing the number and severity of relapses and new MS lesions. There are no easy, like-for-like comparisons between DMDs, and in any case, drugs work differently for each individual. In the end, once your neurologist gives the go-ahead, you can make your own preferred choice, so gather as much information as you can.

As with any drug, it is normal to experience a certain amount of trial and error as you adjust to the therapy. If necessary, it is usually possible to switch drugs. For example, some people with MS do not respond to the beta-interferons, but do to Copaxone.

Before starting DMD therapy

It is important to take the time you need to decide whether or not you are ready to begin DMD therapy. As it's a long-term treatment, you need to have commitment and be confident that you can fit the injection pattern into your lifestyle, including work, leisure and holidays. You also need to weigh up the evidence for and against. Since axonal damage is possible at the outset of MS, many neurologists believe that DMDs should be administered 'the sooner, the better', and routinely offer them at diagnosis. There is an increasing body of evidence that suggests this is important. However, other neurologists caution that since DMDs reduce the relapse rate by only one third, and a fair number of people remain well for years or even decades without any sort of intervention, there is good reason to wait and see how things go. Your particular history of MS and the sort of person you are will also contribute to your decision. Quite a few people find that they initially accept a drug prescription, but then have second thoughts. Perhaps they fear it will confirm their 'sickness'. Often they prefer to try an alternative route first.

One final consideration is whether to go public with your decision to try a DMD. Should you tell those closest to you, or keep it private? If you have children, will you plan to talk with them about needles, injecting, medicinal drugs and illegal drug-taking?

Side effects of DMDs

As these drugs are relatively new, nobody knows their long-term benefits or drawbacks, so it pays to be aware of potential side effects. The most common of these are flu-like symptoms, which affect about 50 per cent of the people using any of the beta-interferons. These manifest as muscle aches, sweating and feverishness often following your first injection, last for about 48 hours and then ease up. Less commonly, they may continue for 3–6 months. You may find that you can manage these side effects by injecting at night and sleeping through them. It can also help to take pain-relieving drugs, such as aspirin, ibuprofen or paracetamol.

Injection site problems are also common with Rebif, Betaferon and Copaxone. Some 50 per cent of patients experience them, but normally in a mild way. For example, the skin often reddens initially, but the effect soon fades. Less commonly, hardened skin and lumpiness develop at the injection site, and can sometimes be painful. With Copaxone a condition called lipoatrophy can develop, whereby fat under the skin is lost in small areas, causing 'craters' or indentations that do not improve with time. This is associated with any injections or use of needles, but tends to affect more women than men. Around 45 per cent of people injecting Copaxone develop lipoatrophy.

Very rarely there are side effects from all the beta-interferons, including changes in menstruation, blood abnormalities, such mild anaemia, liver abnormalities, and a reduction in the white blood cell count. For this reason you will need regular blood tests to check on liver function and blood cell count.

Neurological symptoms, such as a flare-up or increased spasticity after injecting, are also rare, normally resolve within 48 hours, and improve over time.

With Copaxone it is rare but possible to have an allergic reaction, experiencing a tight chest and shortness of breath immediately after injection. This can last from 30 seconds to 30 minutes, but usually happens only occasionally. This allergic reaction can recur randomly at any time, and not solely after the first injection.

Beta-interferons can also provoke an immune response in some people, which means that their immune systems produce antibodies that block or neutralize the drug. Apparently, the fact that neutralizing antibodies develop doesn't necessarily mean the drug isn't working – it is simply working less effectively, particularly when it comes to preventing relapses. Disability development, however, is apparently not affected. Antibodies are much more common with Betaferon (30 per cent) and Rebif (25 per cent) than with Avonex (5 per cent), but often (30–40 per cent of cases) the antibodies disappear given time.

You certainly won't be left in limbo once you start a DMD therapy. You can expect practical support and understanding from your MS nurse from the start, when she or he teaches you how to inject correctly. You will also be given regular review appointments with the MS nurse, and an annual review with your prescribing neurologist. These benefit you personally because they check on your health and level of disability. They also contribute to important research into the long-term effect of DMDs, enabling comparisons to be made between how MS develops over time for patients taking DMDs and those who have not.

Other disease-modifying drugs

A number of therapies that are licensed for other conditions can also be prescribed by neurologists for the treatment of MS.

AZATHIOPRINE (IMURAN)

This is a drug that inhibits the proliferation of all white blood cells and is therefore a general immunosuppressant. All drugs that act in this way usually cause significant side effects, so are not often used.

CORTICOSTEROIDS

Since the 1950s various forms of corticosteroids have been used to reduce the recovery time after an MS relapse. They work as blanket immunosuppressants, forcing the immune system to 'shut up and behave', so to speak. Corticosteroids probably reduce inflammation and are also thought to stop the leakage of harmful blood cells into the central nervous system. When you are struggling through a bad relapse it is such a relief to have it curtailed in any way, despite some side effects. Perhaps you just feel better because something is being done. Whatever the case, corticosteroids and other general immunosuppressive drugs continue to have an effective and specific role in the treatment of MS. They do not provide instant recovery from relapses, nor do they influence the degree of recovery or the actual outcome of the relapse. Neither do they have a long-term effect on overall disability or alter the long-term course of the disease.

Although 80 per cent of neurologists are willing to prescribe corticosteroids for relapses, they tend to do so in only a quarter of cases, and some neurologists never prescribe them at all. Although there is no consensus on their use, everyone agrees that they should not be used indiscriminately. Corticosteroid use is determined by the severity of the relapse and the patient's degree of disability. Generally speaking, only 10–20 per cent of relapses merit corticosteroids.

Corticosteroids are not anabolic steroids used by some athletes for muscle building. The steroids used for MS relapses are synthetic versions of hormones produced naturally in the human body in the adrenal glands. Intravenous methylprednisolone (IVMP) is the most common choice for severe relapses. It is administered into the vein and given in large doses, usually in hospital. Oral dexamethasone is also used.

Among the side effects of corticosteroids are: disturbed sleep, the need to urinate more frequently, a metallic taste in the mouth, an occasional increased heart rate, hot flushes or a red face. Sometimes injection sites can become swollen and painful. Steroids can also affect your mood, especially euphorically, which makes you think your MS is improving.

MITOXANTRONE

This drug is potentially much more toxic than other drugs prescribed for MS and has only been used for the treatment of aggressive relapsing disease. It acts by stopping cells dividing and was developed as an anti-cancer agent. The inflammatory response relies on a rapid increase in immune cells once they get into a tissue in order to kill off invading organisms. So the use of mitoxantrone is akin to chemotherapy in cancer patients and is a sledgehammer approach with major side effects.

INTRAVENOUS IMMUNOGLOBULIN (IVIg)

This therapy has been used in other conditions that involve the immune system and uses a preparation of non-specific human antibodies that has to be injected or infused into a vein. Animal studies have also suggested that it might improve repair processes in the brain. Among MS patients, it appears to reduce MS activity, as viewed from repeated MRI scans, and may produce a small reduction in relapse rate. It continues to be prescribed for MS by some neurologists, even though clinical trials have failed to demonstrate any significant benefit.

MS drugs in development

Although there are numerous clinical trials taking place for new MS therapies, it is worth mentioning a few here because they have either finished clinical trials and are awaiting licensing, or have shown definite promise in early trials.

CAMPATH 1-H (ALEMTUZUMAB)

This is an antibody-based treatment that reduces the number of damaging T-lymphocytes and modifies their activity so that they do not attack the myelin sheath. It has so far been tested in patients with secondary progressive disease, and has a much more powerful effect on the immune system than the beta-interferons. Both the formation of new lesions and the occurrence of relapses were almost completely abolished for 18 months. However, half the patients still showed a progression of disability despite the absence of inflammatory activity in the brain. This is a relatively non-specific approach to changing the immune system, and there are some safety concerns associated with the use of this drug as some patients have developed an overactive thyroid gland. More extensive trials are now under way to see whether early treatment will also stop the progression of the disease.

STATINS (SIMVASTATIN OR ZOCOR)

These drugs, widely used for reducing cholesterol in the blood and thus reducing the occurrence of heart disease, have also been shown to alter the immune response in animal models of MS. MRI scans taken during early clinical trials show that they also reduce the number of new lesions.

TYSABRI (ANTEGREN OR NATALIZUMAB)

This new disease-modifying therapy acts by stopping damaging white blood cells getting across the blood-brain barrier, and has just completed two phase three trials involving more than 2,000 patients over two years. It has been shown to reduce new relapses by 67 per cent and the accumulation of disability (measured using the EDSS scale) by 42 per cent over two years. This makes it roughly twice as effective as the beta-interferons. Applications have now been made to licence the drug for use in MS. It remains to be seen whether this effectiveness continues long-term and whether there are any long-term negative effects of stopping all white blood cell traffic across the blood-brain barrier.

Do these disease-modifying therapies stop the build-up of disability?

The enthusiasm for the currently available disease-modifying drugs, whether started first at diagnosis or at a later stage of MS, must be seen in the light of the disappointing reality that most people taking these drugs continue to have some relapses during treatment, and some have no benefit at all. The latest analysis of the effects of beta-interferons on the progression of disability in MS, after 12 years of treatment, shows little or no beneficial effects. This means that despite slowing down relapses and reducing the formation of new lesions, these drugs do not reduce the likelihood of your MS producing an increasing level of disability with time. The long-term accumulation of symptoms is probably caused by an increasing loss of nerve fibres or axons, so it is thought that drugs that alter the way the immune system works, such as the beta-interferons, are of little use once axon loss (seen as atrophy on a brain MRI scan) reaches a critical threshold. This is now recognized as the stage at which MS becomes secondary progressive.

Research suggests that although nerve fibre damage may be triggered by inflammatory attacks, it then carries on in the absence of inflammation in the nervous system.

Thus, in order to be truly effective, drug treatments that reduce the immune attack must be given as early as possible and should also be complemented with drugs that provide protection to axons and neurons in order to completely stop the progressive nature of MS. The next chapter shows how such 'neuroprotective' treatments are being developed.

Symptomatic therapies for MS

The disability that builds up with MS over a number of years is best managed, where possible, by a multidisciplinary team, and will involve physical therapies and psychological and social interventions, supplemented by medical treatments. The symptoms that are most amenable to treatment are spasticity and bladder dysfunction.

ANTICHOLINERGICS

Failure to store urine in the bladder can be treated by a group of drugs called anticholinergics, in particular Oxybutynin, which acts by inhibiting the detrusor muscle that causes bladder emptying. Failure of the bladder to empty is usually treated by intermittent self-catheterization.

BACLOFEN, DANTROLENE AND TIZANIDINE

Stiffness and spasms, collectively known as spasticity (see page 152), are usually treated with Baclofen (Lioresal) or Tizanidine (Zanaflex), which both work at the level of the spinal cord to reduce muscle tone. Dantrolene (Dantrium) directly targets the muscle fibres and reduces their ability to contract. Spasticity in MS is caused in part by changes in the brain that reduce the ability of the spinal cord circuits to adequately control muscle tone. Managing spasticity is best achieved in a multidisciplinary way: drugs combined with physiotherapy.

MODAFANIL

Fatigue is one of the commonest and most disabling symptoms of MS, but it cannot be successfully treated using drug therapies at present. Clinical trials are currently looking at the use of Modafanil (Provigil), a drug that can be prescribed for narcolepsy, a condition characterized by excessive sleepiness during the day.

PHYSIOTHERAPY

Physiotherapy has been called the cornerstone of treatment for MS, and is beneficial at all stages. It is a hands-on approach based on a thorough knowledge of anatomy and physiology. Physiotherapists work alongside their clients, explaining what is happening and seeking specific ways to help. They have at their fingertips a repertoire of exercises designed to prevent or relieve any movement disorders, to ease mobility, to reduce the possibility of deformity, to relieve neck and back problems that are especially common for people in wheelchairs or in bed, and to assist anyone experiencing difficulty with breathing or swallowing. Some physiotherapists go on to specialize in neuro-physiotherapy, which means that they focus specifically on treating conditions such as MS. They normally work at specialist neurological or rehabilitation centres in big hospitals or out in the community.

Whether working with groups or individuals, a physiotherapist's skill is to use exercises tailored specifically to your individual needs. It's fascinating to experience how creative physiotherapists are at finding different ways to tackle a problem. For example, it is all too easy to slip into walking with a twisted posture or awkward gait as an unconscious compensation for a stiff leg or balance problem. The physiotherapist knows how to systematically exercise limbs and muscles, correct poor posture, improve muscle tone, work towards improved control of movement, and help restore balance and coordination. If fatigue is a problem, it may be that short periods of exercise sandwiched between rest periods can help to increase stamina and endurance.

Physiotherapy will work well if you practise the exercises regularly, keeping a balance between effort and relaxation. One aim of physiotherapy is to maintain mobility and suppleness so that you can remain self-reliant and carry out the functions of everyday living. It is really important to become aware of the range of help a physiotherapist can give – for example, assessing your daily activities at home, work or in leisure time, identifying restrictions and limitations, and finding ways of remedying them. Physiotherapists can also provide suitable equipment for walking or getting around. The benefits are not only physical and practical, but psychological too. It is wonderful to discover a physiotherapist who not only understands the difficulties MS brings and can do something practical about them, but also listens and supports. Physiotherapists have a good reputation among health-care professionals for their counselling approach.

It helps to begin physiotherapy early on, when problems may be only minor, in order to reduce any possible future complications. Initially an intensive training programme of exercises is needed. These may include stretching and weight-bearing exercises to improve your physical condition and help counter spasticity, or aerobic and endurance training to alleviate fatigue. Exercises will always be matched to individual needs. Even if you suffer from severe spasticity, passive exercise, where another person moves your limbs for you, is important each day, as it helps to prevent contractures. A relaxant or painkiller may be necessary for this to be possible, but when the spasticity does ease, the limbs will return to working order much more quickly. Some find it helps to have massage or a bath before physiotherapy exercise, but avoid getting overheated.

Unfortunately, it is rare that anyone gets more than one or two physiotherapy sessions per week under the NHS, and then probably only for a limited period of time. Capitalize on what help is given by continuing to do the exercises at home. Always watch out that you don't go beyond your fatigue threshold. You will certainly gain greater benefit from frequent exercise in small doses. Overtiring yourself in a workout can take days to recover from.

Physiotherapy treatment is normally arranged in Britain by your GP, MS nurse or neurologist on an outpatient appointment basis. Before asking for physiotherapy, think through what problems you have that could benefit from treatment. Also bear in mind that it can be time-consuming and exhausting to wait for transport to and from outpatient clinics, and that this could counteract the benefit of the actual treatment. Occasionally, however, it is possible for a physiotherapist to come to your home to treat you. Physiotherapy is also available at MS therapy centres (see page 287) or may be arranged by your local branch of the MS Society. Of course, treatment is available privately too, but choose a physiotherapist who really enjoys working with people who have multiple sclerosis.

Taking a different path

If you experience an MS remission, it is wonderful to find yourself suddenly free of the symptoms and literally on your feet again. It is as if you have been given your life back, with the added bonus of wisdom and experience gained from juggling your life with MS. This sort of release sometimes comes spontaneously. The inevitable question is 'Why?' If you have just embarked on some sort of treatment when an improvement takes place, you will inevitably credit that treatment positively, but the chances are that it was simply coincidental. Treatments and 'cures' that come out of the blue make a splash in the press and become popular for a while, raising people's hopes. It's understandable that if those with MS believe they have experienced a 'recovery', or 'therapists' get good feedback from some treatment producing dramatic results, they will want to share their good fortune and market whatever it is. This has happened with snake and bee venoms, hyperbaric oxygen therapy, and Cari Loder's 'cocktail' of an anti-depressant, amino acid and vitamin B_{12}. The only way to justify dramatic and unexpected treatments is to submit them to properly controlled trials. This is currently happening with Aimspro, derived from antibodies in goat serum. Of the two trials under way, one is investigating its potential use for secondary progressive MS, and the other for optic neuritis.

What you believe in and fancy is sure to do you far more good than what you are sceptical about. Reading through the rest of this chapter, you are likely to accept a few of the following treatments, therapies and approaches as essential, to consider some as possible, and to dismiss others as quackery. Each has been included because at some time it has been linked with MS. None is a cure; some are generally accepted treatments for MS, and each has its devotees. It is up to you to decide what you want to try. It is likely that at some time and for some people, each may be just the job. It is worth experimenting, provided you remember a few safeguards. People with MS should never push themselves to exhaustion point physically, mentally or emotionally. Only get involved with what you think will suit you personally in terms of health, time, energy and money.

Complementary and alternative therapies

While complementary and alternative treatments can sometimes offer relief from particular MS symptoms (and leave you feeling good afterwards), it is difficult to measure their effectiveness because of the unpredictability and variability of MS. There is little scientific proof, but lots of anecdotal evidence, affirming how much they can contribute to well-being. It is extremely unlikely that any of them will alter the course of MS, and none of them will stop the progression. Any natural remedy takes longer to work than drugs, and at first there may not be any positive indication that it is making any difference at all.

It is important to recognize that complementary and alternative treatments are not necessarily 'safe'. There may be health risks. Natural doesn't necessarily mean harmless. You must be prepared to check out the type of therapy and the qualifications of the therapist. Always make sure you tell the therapist what other medication or treatments you are having.

There is a difference between complementary and alternative medicine and treatments, which may be worth noting. A complementary therapy is used in combination with conventional medicine whereas an alternative one is used in place of it. Every therapy works best when you are relaxed and accepting.

HOMOEOPATHY

Based on the principle that like cures like, homoeopathy is a holistic system of complementary medicine. Ailments are treated with minute doses of a substance that would produce the very symptoms you want to be rid of if it were given in larger doses. In order to determine what will work best, the homoeopath takes time to explore each patient's likes and dislikes, emotional reactions and characteristic responses to life in general. There is never one specific remedy for any symptom: however, there is a remedy suited to any particular patient.

Homoeopathic medicines can be animal, vegetable or mineral in origin, and are so dilute that it is hardly credible there is any potency left. Despite that, results are good but often slow. As these medicines work in animals as well as humans, their positive effects are definitely more than auto-suggestion. Homoeopathic remedies appear to act as triggers for the body's own natural healing forces to kick into action.

There are no large studies of the effects of homoeopathy on MS, and certainly no homoeopath would ever claim to cure the disease. However, a good homoeopath will provide specific remedies for certain MS symptoms, and many people have found them helpful for spasm, bladder problems, double vision and pain. In addition, homoeopathic remedies can minimize the effects of colds, flu or other viral complaints. Although there is no scientific evidence that homoeopathy improves the symptoms of MS, at least there are no side effects.

HERBALISM

Herbal medicines are obtained solely from plants, and contain no added chemicals. From biblical times until early in the twentieth century, herbalism was the main system of healing, an everyday part of life based on treating the whole person. People with MS may find certain herbal treatments helpful, but some can react negatively with conventional drug treatments. For this reason you should always take treatments under medical supervision. (For a reputable herbalist consult the National Institute of Medical Herbalists, see page 296.)

Herbal practitioners vary in the way they diagnose and carry out consultations, and their remedies tend to take longer to work. Herbal treatments never claim to cure

MS, but may alleviate symptoms and promote better health in general.

CANNABIS

For many years now some people with MS have – off the record – reported finding considerable benefit from using cannabis, despite the fact that its use is illegal in the UK. They experience relief from distressing symptoms, such as muscle spasm, especially in the bladder, tremors and pain. Others find no positive effect at all, and a few have had negative reactions, such as impaired posture and balance. Anecdotal evidence shows that cannabis is commonly smoked in cigarettes (with or without tobacco), or vaporized and inhaled, which can cause harm to the lungs. Alternatively it can be added in leaf or resin form to cakes and chocolate or infused in drinks.

As it is still illegal to use or even prescribe cannabis medically, those with MS who would vouch for its therapeutic benefits have long urged for a change in the law. They have argued that cannabis is safe and non-addictive, and insist that it is the only drug that gives them relief, despite the fact that it is a pharmacologically 'dirty' drug, containing a host of ingredients and actions which are promising as well as problematic. Initial surveys carried out to discover what positive contribution cannabis makes to MS have been followed by full clinical trials of cannabis-based drugs to establish which active components in this complex organic compound are beneficial, neutral or harmful. Early results proved inconclusive, despite the enthusiasm of most people with MS on the trial, who were sure they experienced improvements not measurable objectively. However, subsequent analysis over the longer term has proved more positive in relation to muscle stiffness and disability, particularly when tetrahydrocannabinol (THC), the active ingredient in cannabis, is used. Fresh trials are under way, for which there is increasing support from MS charities and groups anxious that people with MS should receive the best and safest treatment for distressing symptoms.

Another avenue of research has shown that cannabis mimics the action of natural cannabis-like chemicals in the brain. This means that it might be possible to manipulate the action of these natural chemicals to make them work harder to reduce pain and muscle spasms without the side effects of cannabis.

Meanwhile, some find the synthetic cannabinoid Nabilone, which can be prescribed, gives reasonably good results, especially for nausea and vomiting, which are not particularly common MS symptoms. The psychological effect of cannabis on people with MS does not appear to be particularly adverse. However, although people with MS who regularly use cannabis report that the real plant produces greater beneficial effects, it is generally recognised as a significant causal factor in mental illness. This risk is greatest for young people predisposed towards it but it can also cause mental health problems for people considered to be at low or no risk.

MASSAGE

Massage is high on the list of complementary treatments for MS in Scandinavian countries, where the populations are convinced that massage is beneficial. A good massage both relaxes and stimulates. It also improves the circulation of the blood, thus aiding the nervous and immune systems to work at peak efficiency. To relieve muscle tension and spasm, an old-fashioned technique called 'cupping', applied either side of the spinal cord, has proved valuable for some people with MS. Massage works well in combination with bathing first. You must expect to feel very tired after it, and may need time to build up a tolerance to its undoubtedly beneficial long-term effects.

REFLEXOLOGY

More than just another form of massage, reflexology divides the body into zones, each of them linked to a key point on one of the feet. By massaging and putting pressure on the appropriate area of the foot, it is possible to treat the problems in the related body zone. Simple and harmless, it often produces surprising results. In MS it seems particularly beneficial for urinary problems and paralysis of the limbs.

EXERCISE

For years many people with MS have fought shy of exercise because so often after exercising they felt more fatigued, and experienced a flare-up of previous symptoms. It is now clear that although exercise can produce an immediate but temporary reaction similar to a relapse, this passes after a short period of rest with no ill effect. Indeed, the overall benefit to general health and MS is very good.

This has been found true for aerobic-type exercise, with sustained and rhythmic activity that raises the pulse and respiration. It is also true for exercise using weights, often practised by people with mobility and balance problems. The most positive result is an increase in leg strength, and there is often some improvement in balance and mobility. When exercising, it is essential to warm up first and cool down afterwards, working gently but persistently in between.

Exercise is important in maintaining general good health, as well as seeming to keep disability somewhat in check. It is particularly helpful to incorporate functional exercises that enable you to practise movements essential to maintain your daily activities.

YOGA

Enthusiasts claim that yoga offers much of specific benefit to MS because it helps maximize energy, tones up the neuromuscular system, affects the immune system positively, improves the function of the glands, builds up resistance to illness and keeps the body supple.

Yoga, particularly the *hatha* form that emphasizes the importance of breathing properly, seems best suited to MS. It includes exercises that help you bend and stretch, squeeze and twist muscles, and work all the joints gently but thoroughly. Yoga movements can be done lying down, sitting on a chair or standing. Many are very simple, the more complex ones being a combination of simpler movements linked together, with careful attention being paid to breath control.

Even if you are unable to move an arm or a leg, allowing yourself to visualize the movement you plan to make and then controlling your breath to give you energy while someone else lifts and moves the limb is also beneficial. It is often difficult with MS to move or hold a position, but just trying to do so often seems to have a retraining effect on the body. It is well worth overcoming any initial reluctance or desire to give up if results are not immediate.

Especially beneficial outcomes for MS are improved flexibility, strengthened muscles, better posture, balance and breathing, and reduced fatigue. Yoga also benefits the internal organs, including the heart and diaphragm, with positive knock-on effects to the digestion and elimination. You learn a fresh awareness of your body, as a whole and to its individual parts, and feel better able to manage your MS.

Yoga combines movement with different types of relaxation, which provide an antidote to the tensions of MS – those that result from the disease itself and those that are a reaction to living with it. There's no doubt that both types of tension can build up to such an extent that people easily get locked into MS. Many people with the disease find yoga teaches them to function fully once more, no longer fragmented, but harnessing the totality of who they are so that they find it easier to cope. It invites you to accept life as it comes and teaches the skills to work in systematic but relaxed ways within the restrictions of the disease or problem area. It gives you new options to replace grim determination and gritting your teeth when faced with a setback. For example, yoga teaches you how to breathe for maximum benefit so that tensions in your body are released and its energy is made fully available. The basis of energy control is knowing how to relax. During relaxation gentle diaphragmatic breathing maintains a continual flow of energy. At other times you may find specific breath control involving the diaphragm invaluable. By taking a strong breath in and then breathing out slowly, you are giving more oxygen to the body and brain, and stimulating energy flow.

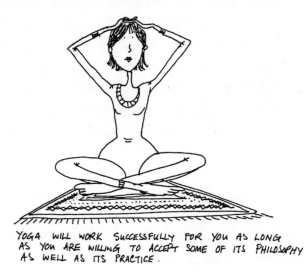

YOGA WILL WORK SUCCESSFULLY FOR YOU AS LONG AS YOU ARE WILLING TO ACCEPT SOME OF ITS PHILOSOPHY AS WELL AS ITS PRACTICE.

Yoga will work successfully as long as you are willing to accept some of its philosophy as well as its practice. It is not a form of treatment, but more a way of taking control of yourself and making a conscious decision to integrate body, mind and spirit into a smoothly functioning whole. If you have time for the whole person approach and are sympathetic to the concept that good health depends on harmony, balance and maintaining natural rhythms, you will discover that yoga has much to offer. It seems to work like a key, unlocking resources in the body that help people live better with MS.

With MS you may find you can fit in easily enough with a mainstream class. Alternatively, look for special remedial yoga classes designed specifically to help you minimize the disabilities of MS and maximize your health potential.

PILATES

The Pilates (pronounced 'pil-ah-tees') approach to exercise for the whole body also offers much of benefit for people with MS. Pilates exercises were originally designed to re-educate the body's neurological reflexes in order to bring about permanent improvement in posture and body alignment. As a holistic method of body maintainance, it prioritizes general fitness and body awareness, which contributes positively to rehabilitation.

Particularly beneficial to MS is that it improves 'core strength', increasing trunk and pelvic stability. Pilates exercises also help improve muscle tone, flexibility and joint mobility, all of which help coordination and ease movement. They also focus on good breathing patterns. Devotees report how much Pilates lowers stress levels.

The exercises are most expertly taught in a Pilates studio, but are also available at health clubs and in informal groups. Many Pilates exercises are creeping into general keep-fit classes.

AROMATHERAPY

Aromatherapists believe that essential oils, extracted from plants, can be absorbed through the skin, travel to the organs, glands and tissues, and seep into the bloodstream and lymph fluid of the body, the results of which may prove healing. In addition, the natural anti-bacterial and anti-viral properties of essential oils appear to increase resistance to infection.

Each essential oil has its own distinctive properties, which have an effect on body, mind and emotions. Many oils seem to serve a multipurpose function, and it makes fascinating reading to discover which favour which part of the body.

By far the best and most effective way of using essential oils is in massage. The action of rubbing is thought to activate the nerve endings and stimulate the circulation of blood at the surface of the skin. In any case, a good massage is in itself relaxing and promotes a sense of well-being. Essential oils can also be added to a warm bath. There they not only come in contact with the skin, but are also inhaled.

Whether or not you accept the theory of aromatherapy, there can be no doubt that it is a very pleasant way of pampering yourself. Even if its beneficial results come merely from enjoying the scent of the oils and the relaxing effects of massage and hot baths, the psychological boost it gives invariably has a positive effect on health.

BIOFEEDBACK

The principle of biofeedback is to make you more aware of particular body functions, and to teach you beneficial ways of controlling them. It involves a certain degree of self-awareness, and employs the techniques of yoga, as well as the technology of modern biofeedback machinery.

More preventative than curative, biofeedback seems to have some value for MS, particularly in relieving stress. The ability to cope with stress depends on recognizing its effects on the body. Many people are never fully aware of them, and struggle on in a permanent state of partial tension. This makes them more prone to psychosomatic problems, which may aggravate MS. Using a biofeedback machine that monitors electrical skin resistance can show people how to recognize body reactions to stress and warn them that they need to relax.

TENS (TRANSCUTANEOUS ELECTRICAL NERVE STIMULATION)

This therapy works by pulsing a low-level electrical current into the body through electrodes placed on the skin. Often self-administered, it is popular among people with MS as a means of reducing and even eliminating pain. The current apparently restricts the transmission of pain impulses, while stimulating the body to produce its own pain-relieving hormones.

TENS units are widely used in hospitals and pain clinics, and are gaining in popularity with physiotherapists. Small, lightweight and portable, they are easy to use and invaluable in controlling many of the pains associated with MS.

HYPERBARIC OXYGEN THERAPY

The term 'hyperbaric' means 'high pressure', and HBO treatment consists of breathing in oxygen under increased pressure through a face-mask while sitting in a specially designed chamber. The resulting raised oxygen content in the blood is thought to benefit several conditions, including MS, though it is generally discounted by medical science. HBO treatment should not be taken by those who suffer from epilepsy or any heart condition.

During the early 1980s sensational media reports of cures or considerable improvement in MS following HBO

treatment started a rush for places, and volunteers under-
went training in the supervision of HBO chambers.
Various trials to assess the true clinical value of the treatment have since been carried out. The results show no
objective and little subjective benefit from HBO.

Hyperbaric oxygen therapy is still available through
most MS therapy centres (see page 287) because some
people with MS do feel they benefit from it. Always check
that there is someone responsible on duty when the chamber is being used, and bear in mind that any positive effect
is unlikely to be lasting.

ACUPUNCTURE

The ancient Chinese practice of acupuncture works on
the principle of there being approximately 800 points in
the body, each of which is linked to an organ. The points
are said to be linked together along lines known as meridians, which work as sort of energy pathways. If the points
remain in balance along their meridian, you enjoy a state
of health. If there is a lack of energy, or an excess of it,
the meridian becomes sensitive and registers a state of
imbalance or illness.

The work of the acupuncturist is to make sure the
meridians have an even flow of energy passing through
them. This is achieved by inserting needles into them to
stimulate specific nerves. The electrical impulses gener-
ated register in the brain, the spinal cord and the affected
area. Needles of pure metal only are used, notably
copper, silver (for a sedative effect) and gold (to stimulate). The acupuncturist knows which meridian to treat
by making a pulse diagnosis at the wrist. This provides

information about the present state of health and may even be predictive.

Acupuncture should not be viewed as a panacea for all ills, but as a treatment that has proved useful over a wide therapeutic range, and one that often combines well with other therapies. Clinical experience shows that it may help to alleviate some symptoms of MS, such as pain, muscle weakness and spasms, tremor, poor balance and coordination, dizziness, urinary tract infections, emotional dysfunction and coldness in the limbs. Too often, however, the relief experienced is only temporary and the symptoms treated are likely to reappear.

HYDROTHERAPY

Water is not only a natural cleansing agent, internally as well as externally, but also provides a supportive environment for exercising.

Hydrotherapy is a form of physiotherapy, where the buoyancy of the water creates an altered, weight-bearing environment that eliminates stresses on joints and helps return motion to the body. This effect is enhanced in salt water.

Although not a fashionable treatment today, hydrotherapy is still much valued by natural therapists. In mainland Europe it is still common for people with MS to be treated with hydrotherapy at clinics in spa towns. In the UK the increasing popularity of day spas should now make it easier to find the specialized treatment here too.

The best spas and hydro centres employ a physiotherapist with expertise in hydrotherapy. Some spas operate non-enclosed flotation pools with saline water,

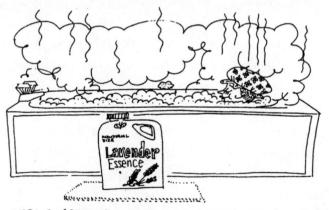

THERE IS GREAT ADVANTAGE IN RELAXING AND UNWINDING IN A BATH, PERHAPS WITH ESSENCES OF PINE AND LAVENDER, SO GOOD FOR THE NERVOUS SYSTEM

which are great places to exercise and relax, provided you can cope with the warm water. (It is common for people with MS to feel weak just from being in warm water, and it can take time for a healthy tolerance to build up. Once that happens, hydrotherapy can energize, as well as create a sense of well-being.)

If private spas are beyond your means, it is worth checking whether your local leisure centre offers hydrotherapy. In some places the Primary Health Care Service has teamed up with Leisure Services to offer people with disabilities exercise programmes on prescription.

Hydrotherapy may be too grand a word for the baths or showers you take at home, but they also contribute to your well-being. The circulation can be stimulated by showering with cold and warm water alternately, but it is also pleasant to relax and unwind in a bath, perhaps with essences of pine or lavender – so good for the nervous system. Tense muscles are eased, and the psychological effect is also very beneficial.

HORSE-RIDING

Many people will probably be surprised to learn that horse-riding can be very therapeutic for those with MS. Indeed, it is particularly encouraged as a form of rehabilitative treatment in Switzerland and Scandinavia. Riding a horse provides gentle exercise for the muscles, improves posture, coordination and concentration, sometimes has a positive effect on spasticity and control of the bladder and bowel, and also provides the benefit of fresh air. The rhythmic movement of the horse seems to mimic human walking, thus stimulating the rider to adjust balance and posture. One good outcome for MS can be an improved gait. Ask local groups offering horse-riding for the disabled if they would welcome people with MS.

Personal support

While family, friends and carers all provide valuable help and support, there are occasions when an outsider or specialist organization may be better equipped to help you through difficult times.

Counselling

Counselling gives you an opportunity to explore in a safe, understanding, professional relationship what it means for you to live with MS. It is difficult to cope with the way MS interferes in your life. If you have the disease, you may find its symptoms so intrusive and frightening that expressing what they are like is the only relief you can get. Yet talking about them as much as you need to will bore and frustrate most people, even those nearest and dearest, and they will lack the impartiality you require. If you don't have MS yourself but are close to someone who has, you too deserve space to express your own reactions and needs. In both instances, talking things through in confidence with a trained counsellor will allow you to face the disease, untap the resources within you and discover the support available from others.

As each person's needs are different, counsellors use their skills to focus on you, the individual, and create the right environment for you to discover in your own way and own time what helps or hinders your coping well with MS. It is to do with unlocking your own inner strengths, which seem to go under wraps when a serious source of stress comes on the scene. You need understanding support before you can accept how normal it is with MS to experience strong emotional reactions, to doubt your own self-worth and to wonder what useful contribution you can still make to the world. Inevitably, you will have to reappraise your relationships at home, at work and socially, and face the fact of a less certain future. Through counselling you can choose to face reality and learn to like yourself. This is a rewarding enough experience in itself. Even more relevant and exciting is the added bonus of an improvement in health. Indeed, it has been said that few diseases are so positively affected by good emotional health as MS.

Some people suppose that only a counsellor who has first-hand experience of MS can counsel someone with the disease. This is not so. The work of the counsellor is not to swap personal experiences of MS – that is the province of a self-help group – but to allow you to discover the facts of MS and how to maximize your life with it. While it is important that you and your counsellor are well informed about MS, your personal reactions to it are the stuff of counselling. Obviously it is essential for every counsellor to appreciate, for example, the strength and pervasiveness of MS fatigue, or the way in which demyelination can affect general mood. However, it is likely that emotional blocks aggravate these symptoms, and resolving the blocks releases energy for healing and coping better with life.

Your GP will be able to refer you to a counsellor or clinical psychologist, or you can make your own arrangements. A counselling session usually lasts for one hour once a week over an agreed period of time. There are many different kinds of counselling, all of them with their merits, but what matters most is that you feel at ease with the counsellor, who should have experience and be in supervision. Trust your instinct after the first interview to decide whether to go ahead with this counsellor on a regular basis, or to have an interview with a different one. The British Association of Counselling and Psychotherapy (see page 290) offers guidelines on how to choose the right sort of counsellor for you.

Hypnotherapy

Hypnosis does not treat symptoms so much as look at the causes of ill health. A fully trained hypnotherapist looks at the whole person and helps you, through hypnosis, to speak freely about your feelings and emotions. When hypnosis works well you will find symptoms may disappear or be reduced as you relax and become aware of your inner self. It is frequently the quickest and most effective method of discovering what pressures you have been under and getting free of them, which would certainly be beneficial if you have MS. On the other hand, you may find it does not work for you, or that it is a technique you regard with suspicion.

Self-help groups

Talking things over with others who have gone through a similar experience is widely acknowledged to be extremely helpful. Self-help is a way of reaching outside yourself, acknowledging your right to get support and believing that others have something to give you. It helps you to live through today and have the courage to want to live tomorrow.

Self-help is not a universal remedy, but just one of many ways of coping with MS. For a long time you may have been on the receiving end of advice and support, but now you can give back as you become actively involved in the process of sharing. In talking about your experience of MS with others who also have it, you give each other mutual support.

Self-help groups are generally small and informal. The focus of the help is on the individual and his or her needs. Who you are and your personal experience of life and MS are what count. It is not always what you say or do not say that makes an impression. The fact that you want to be there to give yourself and others a chance to share is all-important.

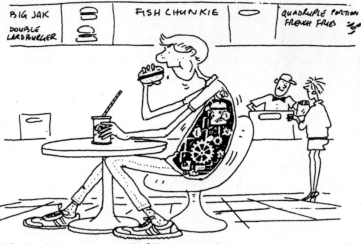

BODIES FED ONLY JUNK FOOD OVERWORK AS THEY STRUGGLE
TO COPE WITH THE LONGER AND MORE COMPLEX PROCESS
OF DIGESTING 'JUNK'

Nutrition and MS

What you eat makes a difference to how healthy you are. Bodies fed only junk food overwork: they struggle to cope with the longer and more complex process of digesting 'junk', and strain to extract the nutrition they require to function well. The healthiest diets are always balanced and do not exclude any one food group. They should include fresh, natural and unprocessed foods: salads, fruits and vegetables, whole grains, nuts and pulses, white fish, chicken, limited amounts of lean red meat, small quantities of dairy products, few eggs and plenty of water. These foods are absorbed easily and broken down efficiently to give you the energy you need.

The best diet for MS must not only be normally healthy, but also compensate for any deficiencies in the nervous and immune systems of the body. The three basic recommendations for improving eating habits are as follows:

- Reduce your intake of saturated (animal) fat.
- Eat five portions of fruit or vegetables each day.
- Include high-fibre starchy foods.

Since research shows that levels of saturated fats are higher and levels of polyunsaturated fats lower than average in people with MS, it is important to follow a low-fat diet. Avoid fatty foods, including the hidden fats in processed foods, such as burgers, crisps and biscuits. Adequate protein is important, as are vitamins and minerals, which occur naturally in fresh fruits, salads, vegetables, nuts, grains and seeds. For example, vitamin C, found in good supply in berries, oranges, kiwis, chillies and green peppers, helps attack viral and bacterial infection. The B vitamins and folic acid are similarly important. Vitamins A and E abound in nuts and seeds, and help protect cells from damage. Minerals, such as calcium, magnesium, selenium and zinc, are also needed. It is best to take your vitamins naturally through the food you eat as they work together in a complex harmony. Swallowing large doses of vitamin supplements, especially single vitamins, can do more harm than good and is also costly.

Although no single diet has been proved to cure MS, there are strong indications that a low-fat diet with additional sunflower oil and vitamins E and A has a very beneficial effect long term. Other diets sometimes recommended are more to do with personal preference, individual taste and circumstantial evidence.

Suggestions for healthy eating

Keep meals simple and low in fat

- Base main meals on brown or basmati rice, whole-meal pasta or jacket potatoes.
- Add a minimal amount of protein in the form of fish, poultry, small portions of lean red meat, an occasional egg (2–3 per week), low-fat cheese, or pulses, such as lentils, beans or soya products (these are not gaseous if you add a little wine to the cooking).
- Eat lots of raw salads and lightly cooked vegetables. Include sprouting seeds, such as alfalfa and mung, which are a rich source of vitamins and minerals.
- Make soups, a comforting way of eating all sorts of vegetables, most of which are rich in plant sugars (prebiotics), which nurture 'good' bacteria in the gut.

Whenever possible use:

- Skimmed or semi-skimmed milk
- Low-fat natural yoghurt
- Margarine or oil high in polyunsaturates, e.g. sunflower or soya
- Low-fat cheese, e.g. cottage cheese, low-fat Cheddar, Edam or Gouda
- Oily fish, such as salmon, mackerel and sardines, at least twice a week
- Skinned poultry and lean meats, grilled, steamed or poached
- Potatoes, baked, boiled, steamed or mashed

- Wholemeal flour products
- Brown rice
- Fresh foods – brightly coloured vegetables are particularly healthy

Avoid rich, fatty, sugary, over-refined and over-processed foods. These include fast foods, most convenience meals, cakes, buns, biscuits and sweets.

Learn to enjoy natural foods. These are items that have not been stripped of their fibre and nutritional content. They include wholegrain bread and cereals.

Increase your fluid intake, especially of pure water. To maintain optimum health we should all drink 1.5–2 litres a day.

Fat in the diet

A diet low in saturated fats is strongly advised for those with MS. Dietary fat is *probably* the single most important nutrient associated with the disease. Epidemiological studies since the 1950s have indicated a strong association between dietary fat and MS, while foods rich in polyunsaturates are demonstrably helpful for MS. So it really does make sense to watch your fat intake and thereby boost your chances of keeping MS in check.

Saturated fats, often called hard fats because they are solid at room temperature, include butter, lard and coconut oil. It is generally accepted that saturated fats are linked with cancer and heart disease. Less widely known is that there is a correlation in certain countries between a high level of saturated fat in the diet and an increased incidence of MS. Saturated fats actually are unnecessary in the diet, as the body has no problem in producing them by converting other food sources.

Unsaturated fats, which are soft or liquid at room temperature, come in two types: monounsaturated fats, such as olive oil, and polyunsaturated fats, found in fish and plant foods, which contain essential fatty acids (EFAs). These are indeed essential for the healthy functioning of the body, the development of the central nervous system and the growth of nervous tissue, as well as keeping cell membranes fluid and flexible. In MS they help not only to maintain healthy tissue, but may also improve our ability to repair damage to myelin. Western diets are often relatively deficient in EFAs because the body does not create polyunsaturates for itself – it relies on the food you eat to provide them. Any deficiency in essential fatty acids has a negative effect on the function and maintenance of the body.

Essential fatty acids can be divided into two groups significant for MS: linoleic acid, which is found especially in the oils of nuts and seeds, and gamma linolenic acid, present in leafy vegetables, evening primrose oil and fish oils. People with MS often have low levels of both of these EFAs in their blood cells and body fluids, and also tend to have an unusual pattern of EFAs in their blood anyway. Clinical trials have shown how that pattern tends to become normal within a year if you follow a diet rich in polyunsaturates.

Once any EFA deficiency is made good, people with MS generally experience a positive effect on their MS. Upping consumption of polyunsaturates appears to produce a clear reduction in the frequency, duration and severity of MS relapses, especially for people with early relapsing-remitting MS and little or no disability at the start of the treatment. In addition, there seems to be a mild overall benefit, with less accumulation of disability. There is additional evidence from other auto-immune diseases that the use of a low-fat diet and EFA supplements, such as sunflower oil, is beneficial. It therefore seems wise to include good quantities of polyunsaturates in your diet, perhaps with added oil supplements as recommended by NICE, to slow down the disabling effects of MS. There is no consensus as to how much supplementary oil should be taken. It would seem that the addition of at least 20g of sunflower oil per day is of positive value.

Good sources of essential fatty acids

Oils made from sunflower, safflower, soya, corn, grapeseed, blackcurrant, evening primrose, borage. These can be used in salad dressings, for cooking, spread on toast, or simply swallowed neat.

Oil supplements can boost your intake of EFAs. Opt for those including fish oils.

Nuts and seeds, especially walnuts, brazils, almonds, peanuts and peanut butter, sunflower seeds, pumpkin seeds, sesame and poppy seeds.

Green-leafed vegetables (the darker the better), especially broccoli and salads. (They're also found to a lesser extent in green peppers, beansprouts and carrots.)

Wheatgerm, the seeds of wheat, is found in bread or may be bought separately and added to cereals and savoury recipes.

Fruits, including tomatoes.

Soyabeans, and their products.
Oily fish, such as cod, mackerel, salmon and sardines.
Poultry, such as chicken, turkey and guinea fowl.

A word of caution: don't just add foods rich in essential fatty acids to your diet without making other dietary adjustments at the same time. You must reduce your intake of saturated (animal) fats so that your overall consumption of fat is not unhealthy. (The recommended daily amount is 70g for women, and 90g for men.) In addition, since saturated fat competes with essential fatty acids and reduces their beneficial effects, it's crucial to limit saturated fat to let the 'good fats' win.

The role of antioxidants

Antioxidant nutrients – vitamins A, C and (especially) E, richly available in fruit and vegetables – are vital in combating oxidative stress, which occurs when substances within the body react and cause damage to cells. Antioxidants work their magic by converting these damaging substances into harmless ones, such as water and oxygen. Eating protective nutrients found in natural foods, such as fruit and vegetables, together with increased consumption of essential fatty acids, therefore provides an important balance.

Exercise and diet

Any diet works best when it is combined on a daily basis with exercise. This may be difficult when you have MS, but even 10 minutes a day is beneficial. The lymph fluid, which carries immune cells around the body, keeps on the move because of muscular contractions provided by movement. Even if you cannot jog or do aerobics, gentler types of exercise and massage can be effective too. Exercise will also aid the digestion, enabling you to benefit fully from the food you eat.

Dietary allergies and MS

It is possible to experience MS-type symptoms because of allergy problems, and this has been the catalyst for several much-publicized diets designed to improve MS. For example, the Swank Diet is low in fat and cuts out sugar, while the Evers Diet recommends huge quantities of fresh fruit and vegetables, grains and a very low fat intake. Other diets limit you to eating only raw foods, having only liquid, or restricting protein or fructose. The MacDougall and Rita Greer diets are basically gluten-free, low in sugar, low in saturated fat and abundant in fruits, vegetables and pulses. In both cases they were devised by people who maintained that they had recovered from their MS symptoms as a direct result. Although some people with MS will have allergy problems as well as MS, generally speaking it makes little sense to latch on to one particular diet unless it obviously does you good.

There is ample evidence that some people with MS are especially sensitive to certain foods, including dairy products, yeast, mushrooms, fermented products (such as vinegar), sugar, potatoes and tea. If you think you may be allergic to any foods or chemicals, you should get properly tested. This usually begins with a total or cleansing fast, then various foods are reintroduced in order to eliminate any you may be allergic to.

Alcohol and MS

Although widely regarded as one of life's great pleasures, alcohol also has its drawbacks. It adversely affects the central nervous system, and also suppresses the immune system. Excessive drinking progressively weakens the immune system, making those with MS more susceptible to attacks.

'Sensible drinking' is defined by the Department of Health as 3–4 units per day for men and 2–3 units for women. (One unit equals a small glass of wine or half a pint of beer.) However, some people with MS find that they have to reduce the number of drinks they have because they become 'legless' much sooner than they used to. If alcohol has such an effect on your MS symptoms, you should avoid it or strictly limit your drinking.

Remember that alcohol cannot be consumed if you are taking certain medications, so always check with your GP or pharmacist.

Smoking and MS

As so many doctors shrug their shoulders when asked if it is all right to smoke if you have MS, they obviously operate on the principle that anything that gives pleasure and temporary relief is worthwhile, even if it actually does harm. However, there is ample evidence that smoking is harmful in general, and that it can have particularly negative effects on MS.

When you smoke you inhale carbon monoxide, which forms a fixed and irreversible combination with the haemoglobin in your blood. This has two effects: first, the blood thickens and the circulation of it is reduced; then the blood can no longer take up oxygen so easily, and you experience breathlessness as a result. This is bad news on two counts because the central nervous system requires healthy blood circulation, and if MS has reduced your mobility, your breathing capacity has already been lowered. The end result is that you are more likely to suffer from bronchitis and pneumonia.

Tobacco contains a number of poisons, one of which is nicotine. This has a powerful effect, interrupting the transmission of messages along the nerve pathways. Another of the poisons is cyanide – not produced in dangerous quantities, but enough to cause some negative effect.

Smoking also has a pronounced effect on the peripheral nerves, putting them under pressure. For example, if you already have trouble with opening the bladder, the problem will be aggravated because smoking strengthens the bladder's sphincter, the muscle responsible for keeping the bladder shut.

Financial help

You may be entitled to some form of financial assistance because of difficulties caused by MS. Many of the organizations listed in the Useful Addresses section (see page 284) can give further information about this.

Possible benefit entitlements

- Access to Work Grant
- Attendance Allowance (for the over 65s)
- Council Tax Benefit
- Disability Living Allowance (with care and mobility components)
- Housing Benefit (if you rent your home)
- Incapacity Benefit
- Independent Living Fund
- Income Support (for the under 60s), or Minimum Income Guarantee
- Job Seekers Allowance
- Sickness Benefit
- Social Fund
- Statutory Sick Pay
- Working Tax Credit

People with a disability and their carers are entitled to have their health and social care needs assessed. Services can include health care, help in your home and residential care. If appropriate, the Department of Health and Social Services will offer you a package of support. You should receive details of your specific care plan in writing and have the opportunity to discuss it. This is usually organized through the social services department of your local authority.

Possible support entitlements

- Home help for such things as cleaning and shopping
- Disability equipment and adaptations to your home

- Transport services
- Day centres to give you or the person who cares for you a break
- Respite and residential care

Once your care plan and the services to meet your assessed needs have been agreed, you can choose whether to have them provided by your local authority or to receive direct payments to buy them. Using the direct payments route allows you choice and control over the type of support you need.

Carers may also receive support, for their job is very important. They too can ask for a local authority assessment so that their own needs as carers are met, and they can continue in their caring role that makes such a difference to those they care for. (See *The Carers and Disabled Children Act 2000*, available from the DHSSPS.)

Getting the care you need

We often learn what we need or want by discovering what we don't want or like. This holds as true for MS care as everything else.

MS multidisciplinary care

At last the need for a coordinated programme of care for people with multiple sclerosis is being addressed through the concept of specialist MS multidisciplinary teams. The vision certainly exists on paper, is widely backed and marks a shift towards a more holistic approach to MS. A few multidisciplinary teams and centres already exist and offer a sterling service, but there is an urgent need for more. Too often people with MS and their carers are left in limbo, when what they need is seamless and coordinated care to tackle the daily challenges they face.

Recent significant changes have improved the care of people with MS. Increasingly, the compound effect of the 'new breed' of neurologists, some of whom specialize in MS, the growing ranks of specialist MS nurses, and the success of 'tools', such as disease-modifying drugs, that help manage MS symptoms, spells greater confidence all round. Long-term conditions are no longer considered incurable, and those who have them are increasingly regarded as experts in managing their disease. While all this is commendable, there is no room for complacency. The complexity and disabling potential of MS demands quality care delivered speedily and compassionately. Anything less simply will not do.

Although GPs are the natural first choice for support and care, MS nurses are becoming the key MS care workers in the United Kingdom. Fortunately, more are being funded, so you are likely, but by no means certain, to be able to turn to a nurse with specialist MS skills. Sometimes an MS nurse has to cover a wide area single-handed, but in large cities with a hospital-based MS centre several MS nurses may work in a team, each of them contributing an additional skill, such as counselling or palliative care. In addition to supporting you and your family, MS nurses keep abreast of the latest research into the disease, educate where necessary, and network with other health-care professionals. They usually work closely with general practitioners, neurologists and other nurses, as well as physiotherapists, occupational and speech therapists, continence advisers, psychologists and counsellors, social workers and dietitians, as required. They can point you in the right direction for wheelchairs or other aids for living and communicating. In a sense, they will help you to 'create' your very own multidisciplinary team to meet your current MS need. Such teamwork benefits you and also increases their confidence in making a meaningful difference when it comes to MS. In one large UK city a similar role of coordination is being undertaken by a designated MS social worker. Such champions are needed, and they, in turn, need our backing.

Rehabilitation, recovery and hope

Rehabilitation is difficult to put in a box, to package as a product like a pill or an injection. Although rehabilitation depends on knowledge of science, psychology and medicine, and its outcome is visible and measurable, it is not an exact science. It is more than getting something sorted: it seeks to develop your potential. Rehabilitation arises from who we are with MS, and what we are willing or unwilling to tolerate and invest in. It focuses on what we find the greatest handicap with MS, perhaps a particular symptom or a lack of independence. We must spell out what we really want help with. Onlookers, including carers, can make calculated guesses about what is significant, but theirs is an external judgement. Whoever is involved in your rehabilitation − consultant, nurse, occupational therapist, physiotherapist, partner or friend – achieves results only with your active participation.

Recovery is a strange word to use in connection with multiple sclerosis, yet the body has powers of recovery we rarely pay attention to. Think of when you're under the weather: often the best thing to do is wait and let your body recover in its own time. It is important to learn when to hold back and when to move on – and never to cry wolf. Recovery is rarely an all-or-nothing experience: it's about accepting what we cannot do in order to focus on what we can still do. It will always include episodes of pain and struggle, but is also marked by times of inner peace.

We all need hope, no matter how small and fragile its flame, to illuminate our journey with MS. People who love and support us encourage us to hope. Hope becomes contagious in a supportive environment, where self-help and cooperation are encouraged, and champions and advocates are welcomed for the good of all. In such an environment there is no need to be 'fully recovered', simply recovering hopefully.

Trends in MS research

Back to the puzzle

Those of you living with MS do not need to be told that it is a complex condition. As this book demonstrates, it is a giant jigsaw puzzle – an analogy often used to explain why research has not produced a cure, or even a treatment that significantly slows the progression of the disease in most people. The fact that the correct pieces have yet to be put in place is the usual explanation for this apparent lack of progress towards a better treatment. But the jigsaw that is MS is not one of those with thousands of pieces of sky all looking the same, but is one of those puzzles in which every piece is full of intricate detail and needs to be very carefully matched with the adjoining pieces. And, of course, it is a four-dimensional puzzle because MS changes with time in each individual. The placing of one new piece will probably make it necessary to re-evaluate the way previously inserted pieces were arranged. What some of those pieces are and how they fit together, or at least appear to belong in roughly the same area, are explored in this chapter, which looks at what current research tells us about MS.

The sort of questions that people with MS want answers to are simple. However, because the human body is so complex, and the brain is the most complex part of it, even the names of the various branches of science involved in MS research sound baffling. The pieces of the jigsaw thought to be at the centre of the puzzle involve the fields of basic and clinical immunology and the biology of myelin-producing cells and neurons. The disciplines of neurophysiology, virology, genetics and psychosociology, plus rehabilitation and ways of improving diagnosis, complete the list of research components. Until the cause of MS becomes clear, everyone with an interest in the disease, personal as well as professional, is driven to return to the jigsaw again and again, just to see if they can fit in a piece of the puzzle that no one else has noticed – the piece that will make all the difference.

Everyone wants a cure for MS. If you live with it, more practical answers become urgent when you find your life disrupted by its symptoms.

What do scientists think MS is?

There is general agreement that MS appears to be a type of auto-immune disease triggered by environmental factors in individuals with a genetic susceptibility. An auto-immune disease is one in which the body's immune system mistakenly attacks its own healthy cells or tissues instead of a foreign invader, such as a virus or bacterium. In MS the attack by the immune system is thought to concentrate on myelin and/or the cells that produce it, the oligodendrocytes. Although dysfunction of the immune system may be the cause of the inflammation and destruction of myelin, the possible involvement of environmental triggers and genetic susceptibility mean that MS has to be considered a multifactorial disease – in other words, a disease that occurs only when a certain combination of factors are brought together in an individual person. It is important that each factor is investigated separately in order to find out its role in causing MS. Once the individual parts of the picture are in place, we can begin to study how together they could lead to the development of MS. The initial triggers that set off other auto-immune conditions, such as insulin-dependent diabetes and rheumatoid arthritis, also remain unknown, but this does not mean that they cannot be successfully treated.

Why is the cause of MS still unknown?

The quick answer is that MS is one of the most complex conditions that can affect the human body. It shares this complexity with other diseases thought to be auto-immune in nature. It is likely that the condition is triggered long before disturbing neurological symptoms become apparent. Then, once the triggering agent has done its work, the disease may carry on in the complete absence of that agent, which would now no longer be detectable in the body. Unless it leaves behind incriminating fingerprints, it is very difficult detective work indeed to establish the trigger. So in order to discover the causative agent it may be necessary to study large numbers of people who carry susceptibility genes but do not yet have symptoms of MS.

The enormity of this task becomes clear when you realize that millions of people in the UK alone may carry such genes. In addition, scientists are still not sure what they should be looking for in people who carry these genes. The painstaking process of unravelling MS therefore continues to involve the coordinated efforts of researchers from many different scientific disciplines. This is also why the majority of MS research is directed towards finding out how the immune system damages the nervous system, so that new treatments can be designed to stop this happening. Knowing the causative agent that triggers MS is thus not an absolute requirement for developing new treatments that will effectively stop the devastating symptoms. It is, however, the Holy Grail in scientific terms of any research into a disease.

Types of MS research

It is impossible in this book to provide an exhaustive account of all the MS research around the world, but this section summarizes the broad topics of research and reveals how specific problems are being investigated.

Biomedical research

The primary aims of biomedical research are to understand what causes MS, why the immune system damages the nervous system, how to prevent it and how to repair the damage. The biology of myelin, how it is made and why it is destroyed in MS, is one of the major areas of basic research relevant to MS. As more is understood about myelin, it seems increasingly likely that damaged myelin may be repaired or regenerated (remyelination). Armed with a knowledge of how the nervous system can make new myelin-producing cells, researchers will be able to design treatments that improve the body's capacity for repairing the damage.

The other major area of current MS research is in immunology. Much of this research focuses on understanding how auto-immunity occurs. In MS it is vital to understand more about the attacking cells and how they move from the blood into the nervous system. How do such destructive cells cross the blood-brain barrier? If they could be stopped from getting into the central nervous system in the first place, MS would be prevented in people at risk of developing the disease. Alternatively, if the destructive cells do slip through, another preventive measure would be to stop them from attacking myelin. The idea of exterminating the attacking cells before they cause demyelination may sound like something in a child's video game but it is one option. Another option is to alter the immune response to convince it not to attack myelin, which would also lead to new treatments for MS.

Data from epidemiological studies suggests that some environmental factor may be important in triggering MS. This has always been thought likely to be a virus, although no single virus has so far been linked with MS. If there were a virus, then a vaccine could be developed. Advances in genetics are showing us that some diseases are caused by a single defective gene. This is not considered to be likely for MS, but there is sufficient evidence to suggest that a complex combination of certain normal genes makes a person prone to developing the disease. A positive outcome would be if those susceptible to developing MS later in life could be identified genetically, especially during childhood. New therapeutic strategies could then be developed to prevent the onset of MS.

MS tissue studies

MS is a condition unique to human beings, so the starting point for any scientific investigation into how to reverse the damage it causes to the central nervous system is to study the actual tissue that MS has damaged, which is the brain and spinal cord of people who have or had MS. There are two different approaches to this. The advent of the MRI scanner has allowed investigations to be carried out on the living intact nervous system of people affected by MS, and ever more sophisticated scanners are being developed in order to improve this technique. However, the other important way of looking at the cells and molecules involved in causing the damage and carrying out repair is to study the very tissue that MS has damaged.

A good example of how this is achieved is the UK MS Tissue Bank, set up in 1998 on the Charing Cross Hospital Campus of Imperial College in London. It coordinates the donation and collection of MS and non-MS brain and spinal cord tissue from people who wish to bequeath them to MS research after they die. The tissues are then distributed to research scientists worldwide, and to date over 60 different research projects have benefited.

The tissue bank is a vital resource for MS research, and those who agree to bequeath tissues after they die are providing a priceless legacy to help research into better treatments for future generations.

Research into improving diagnosis

MRI (magnetic resonance imaging) scanning is by far the most important advance in diagnosing MS and studying it in the living patient. MRI scanners are safe to use on a regular basis, and sensitive enough to pick out areas of lesions in the brain and spinal cord. They act like a window, allowing researchers to view what is happening in the central nervous system. Thus, they are helpful (but not always absolutely necessary) for diagnostic purposes, and invaluable for monitoring the results of clinical trials. It is now possible to see whether a new treatment is having an effect on the number of new areas of damage that develop. Scanners also allow the monitoring and study of neuron damage (axon loss) by measuring subtle changes in the volume of certain areas of the brain and spinal cord.

When MRI scanning was first used it was expected that close observation of inflammation and demyelination would reveal a definite correlation between what was seen on the scans and the actual disability suffered by the person with MS. This has not proved to be the case. The number and size of lesions does not always correlate with the visible symptoms. However, by using new technology such as MR spectroscopy, MRI scanners can detect not only very early changes in myelin and identify lesions at different stages of development, but can also focus in on damage that extends beyond the myelin. There is a strong likelihood that the severity of disability that accompanies the primary progressive form of MS, and occurs in the secondary progressive phase, is the result of axon loss, in addition to the regular damage to the myelin sheath. Further research is being carried out to find out how to study this axon loss in greater detail, and also how to identify areas of repair, which is not yet possible using available methods. Being able to measure repair would allow neurologists to monitor the effectiveness of new drug treatments that are thought to work by stimulating the repair processes.

Research into symptom control

Not all research is aimed at understanding and preventing the damage to the nervous system. If you are affected by MS, you will also need drug treatments that alleviate some of the symptoms you are experiencing. Although the disease process itself may not be altered, the quality of life with MS may be improved. Symptomatic treatments include a range of drugs and simple surgical procedures. The problems they correct are often not unique to MS, so new treatments for certain symptoms may be developed by researchers working in other specialities. A good example of this is the current search for drugs that may alleviate the considerable problem of fatigue in MS. Drug development in this area has been stimulated largely by the problems associated with chronic fatigue syndrome and narcolepsy, and new treatments developed for these conditions are now licensed for use or are entering clinical trials for MS.

It is natural that people with MS want to find ways of walking better or controlling their hand movements, and research into how this can be achieved is ongoing. Impaired movement can arise for a number of different reasons: weak muscles, spasticity, loss of coordination, lack of balance and/or impaired sensation. Anti-spasmodic drugs, muscle relaxants or anti-inflammatory drugs, along with physiotherapy and yoga, are common and effective ways of helping people with MS to keep supple, coordinated and mobile. These approaches have been refined by using electronics to determine what causes muscle weakness. This can be due to actual weakness, or to the fact that messages to the muscles are not getting through. Electronic muscle stimulation devices, together with appropriate exercises to make muscles work, are found to be beneficial. Other areas of symptomatic research include bladder and bowel disturbances, tremor, sexual dysfunction, cognitive disturbance and some kinds of pain.

Psychosocial rehabilitation and research

Why must MS keep interfering with what you want to do in life? What can make life better? Research into how best to live with the disease and what type of support people with MS and their families need is vital too. This is achieved in two ways: through research projects that survey general and specific needs, and also through individual practical support.

Psychosocial research projects look at ways of

improving the quality of life with MS – physically, emotionally, socially and at work. Researchers work alongside people with MS and their families, helping them to assess priorities, particularly when resources are limited.

Rehabilitation is too often thought of as offering only physical help. In fact it is best tackled via a team approach in which each practitioner – the MS nurse, occupational therapist, pharmacologist, physiotherapist, neurologist and continence adviser – has a sensitive understanding of the psychology of living with a chronic disease. One difficulty with any treatments that aid rehabilitation (from a scientific perspective at least) is how to evaluate their true effectiveness. For example, if the usefulness of physiotherapy or yoga is being tested, it is hard to fake the treatment, as would be necessary to create a control group. This is done to prevent the 'placebo effect' (the power of suggestion) skewing the results. Inevitably, with a chronic disease such as MS, depression is relatively common, so any ray of hope, improved support or increase in activities and interests will do a lot to boost morale and may appear to bring about a neurological improvement too. It takes time and the discipline of double-blind testing to show whether any physical improvement is genuine.

From the perspective of people with MS, anything that might ease the grip of the disease is worth a try: any practical improvements, no matter how minor, are worth pursuing. These include remaining as comfortable and pain-free as possible, maintaining an optimal level of independence, being able to get where you want to go, retraining for new jobs or pastimes, and not suffering discrimination because of MS. It's also important to have access to therapies that enhance well-being physically, mentally, emotionally and spiritually. It makes a world of difference to people with MS and all who care for and about them that treatments, such as physiotherapy, and services, such as continence advice, sexual counselling, speech therapy and cognitive rehabilitation, are readily available. It is a simple matter of human dignity: to be enabled to take responsibility and make a contribution.

Major questions in biomedical research

Here we look in greater detail at some of the areas that biomedical researchers are investigating in an attempt to solve some of the great mysteries about MS.

Is MS caused by nature or nurture?

As in the past, so today every area of scientific and medical knowledge is eagerly scanned, no longer simply for pointers to a cause and cure for MS, but more for further pieces of the puzzle. Epidemiological research is the study of populations for certain kinds of data: who they are in terms of race and origin; where they live in terms of latitude, environment and climate, and how they live in terms of livelihood, hygiene, nutrition and diet. Such studies can focus on a particular group of people over a limited time period, or an extended (or longitudinal) survey covering several generations. It is epidemiological investigation that unearths clues and suggests directions to be followed up by researchers in other disciplines. The everyday sort of questions that we ask about MS fall within the sphere of epidemiologists. Who gets MS? Is there an equal chance of getting MS irrespective of where you live? Does it make any difference if you are born and grow up in one region, then move to another in adulthood? When do people get MS? What links are there between MS and the environment?

Epidemiology has already shown that patterns of MS vary from one racial group to another, and thus paves the way for analytical research to be done by geneticists. Epidemiologists have found evidence suggesting the involvement of an environmental factor in MS, comparisons between the high prevalence of MS in the cool temperate zones, most especially in the north and among people of Nordic stock, and its apparent absence near the equator and poles, and documentary evidence from areas with a high MS population. The cause is likely to be a combination of genetic make-up and where we live, but proof remains elusive. It has been suggested that the migration patterns of particular racial groups that carried susceptibility genes have an important influence on regional variation. However, there are some examples where this does not seem to be the main determinant affecting susceptibility. For example, migration studies show that the risk of developing MS in a single ethnic group varies according to the place of residence during a critical period of childhood. The low frequency of MS in Africans increases substantially for first-generation descendants raised in the UK. This indicates an important role for environmental factors. The finding that people in Tasmania run a six-fold greater risk of developing MS than people in the Northern Territories of

Australia, despite a similar mix of racial backgrounds, also argues for an important environmental effect.

Other evidence documented by epidemiologists is the personal experience of people with MS – how they cope, the effects of MS on their lifestyle and the typical progression of the disease. This type of information enables doctors and health-care specialists to understand better how to manage MS and best support those with it.

WHAT IS THE ROLE OF GENETICS IN MS?

Why me? Why my son or daughter, my brother or sister, my mother or father? Why do some people get MS and others not? What are my chances of getting MS if I am related to someone with it? Are the genetic factors of MS passed on from generation to generation?

To answer the last question first, the news is good: children of MS parents have a 99 per cent likelihood of staying free of the disease. MS is not hereditary. What we do inherit is a genetic make-up that makes us more or less susceptible to developing MS. This is not unique to MS: susceptibility to developing many conditions is determined by our genes. Rather than causing it to happen, this merely sets the scene for it to develop. However, only some people predisposed to MS will develop it. In addition, an environmental factor, still unspecified, has to be added to the genetic predisposition.

There is little doubt that there is an increased risk of developing MS when other family members are already affected. A genetic contribution to the possibility of developing MS has been made clear by the study of affected twins. If there were no genetic contribution, identical (monozygotic) and non-identical (dizygotic) twins would have an equal chance of getting MS. However, this is not the case: if one twin is affected by MS, there is about a 35 per cent chance that an identical twin will also be affected. This risk drops to around 5 per cent if the twin is non-identical. If you have a non-twin brother or sister with MS, the likelihood of your also developing MS drops further to just over 2 per cent. The risk of developing MS in the population as a whole is around 0.1 per cent. So it is now very clear that MS is not an inherited disease because no families have been found so far in which MS is directly inherited. This is in contrast to the findings of research on Parkinson's, Alzheimer's and motor neurone disease, where a small percentage of cases have been shown to be the result of a direct gene mutation passed through the family.

At least eight different studies have now been completed by geneticists who have been studying the entire human genome in families affected by MS for evidence of MS susceptibility genes. Their conclusions are that MS is a true polygenic condition, which means that many genes make a small contribution to an increased susceptibility, and only when all occur together in an individual person is there a significant increase in their chance of developing MS. The majority of the genes that have a small effect on susceptibility are involved in controlling the immune system in some way, a fact that is not entirely unexpected, considering the theory that MS is an autoimmune condition in which control of the immune response is faulty.

It is important to point out that the genes that increase

susceptibility to MS are not mutations of the sort that lead to the wrong type of protein being produced, as is the case with cystic fibrosis, for example. They are natural variations in genes and are present in large numbers of people in the general population. Genetics research has thus provided facts that at least put you in the picture and enable you to make intelligent choices, even though you might find those facts alarming.

ARE VIRUSES INVOLVED IN CAUSING MS?

There is sufficient epidemiological evidence to suspect that MS could be initiated by a virus. The search for an infectious agent, virus or bacterium that could cause MS has been going on for almost a century. We know that some common viruses, such as measles and rubella, can enter the brain and cause inflammation and demyelination, but this is usually completely reversible and does not recur. There are several viruses that cause conditions similar to MS in animals, such as canine distemper in dogs and Theiler's virus in mice. Indeed, the latter is used as an animal model of MS because it causes persistent neurological deficits, and the tissue damage is similar to that in some forms of MS.

The way most common viruses work is to infect cells, replicate and cause host cell death before they are attacked and destroyed by the body's natural defence mechanisms. This also causes inflammation-mediated tissue damage due to the immune response. A virus might act directly on the central nervous system and infect myelin-producing cells, the oligodendrocytes, or it might act more indirectly. Examples of indirect action might include a virus triggering off an auto-immune response, or a viral agent causing non-specific injury to the central nervous system. On the other hand, the immune system may mistakenly attack the brain because some component of the nerve-insulating myelin sheath closely resembles the virus, or because the virus itself persists in a dormant state in the brain. All these scenarios have been demonstrated in other viral-induced diseases. However, the infecting virus is usually identifiable, either because virus particles can be found in the infected tissue, or because the immune system produces antibodies against the virus. There have been many reports claiming that virus particles are present in MS tissues, but none of these findings have been verified by other scientific studies. Elevated levels of antibodies are indeed found in the blood of people with MS, but they are against a broad range of infectious agents, many of which are very common childhood infections. This is taken to indicate an enhanced immune response in general in people with MS.

It remains possible that common viral infections that occur in people who are genetically susceptible to MS and have defective immune system control mechanisms could be responsible for some cases of MS. It also remains possible that a persistent, non-replicating virus infection, which has not yet been identified, is recognized by the immune system as a target for an inflammatory response in MS. However, these possibilities must remain conjecture until supported by scientific evidence. More recently, the common human herpes virus-6 (HHV6) and the *Chlamydia pneumoniae* bacterium were suggested to have a role in causing MS, but the scientific evidence was not reproduced in further studies. So in conclusion, no one virus has been found to be the obvious culprit, but the possible role of viruses cannot yet be put to sleep. Clearly, research must continue in order to find out how viruses could be involved.

Why and how does the immune system attack the nervous system in MS?

The immune system is a highly complex system of defence against infection. The key to the ability of this system to work rapidly and efficiently are two types of white blood cells: T- and B-lymphocytes. When we become infected by a foreign body, T-lymphocytes are stimulated to start the immune response, and this usually leads to the production of antibodies by the B-lymphocytes. The warning that an invader has breached our defences occurs when T-lymphocytes detect *antigens*. These are complex molecules on the surface of cells, usually, but not always, small parts of proteins, which the immune system either recognizes as 'self' and ignores, or fails to recognize and so attacks the cells as alien. Virtually all aspects of immune system regulation are investigated in MS research because a defect at any one of the stages could lead to inflammation. Until researchers can explain in detail how the complex regulatory processes of the immune system are damaged in MS, there will be no sure way of treating the damage. The guiding principle of immunotherapy must be to maintain a balance between controlling the disease and not stopping the immune system from fighting infection normally. The next two sections discuss some of the advances that have been made.

THE AUTO-IMMUNE HYPOTHESIS OF MS

A vital function of the healthy immune system is to recognize itself and not destroy its own tissue by mistake. Normally this occurs due to something called 'tolerance'. During the early years of its development the immune system is shown a large number of proteins and other molecules from the body that it learns to recognize as 'self'; it becomes tolerant to these proteins. In auto-immune diseases something triggers the cells of the immune system to recognize one or several proteins as 'foreign', when they are in fact 'self'. The immune system then sets out to destroy any cells that have the protein(s) present on their surface. In an auto-immune disease such as myasthenia gravis, where only one 'self' protein is recognized as 'foreign', it is easy to find out which protein is involved because everyone with the disease will be making antibodies against that one protein. This is easy to detect in the blood using a very simple laboratory test. In MS unfortunately, matters are not so clear cut. Everything tells researchers that the target of the faulty immune response is something on the surface of the myelin sheath and/or the oligodendrocyte. Yet so far there does not appear to be any one protein that the immune system is targeting. The protein could even be different between individuals with MS, or several proteins could be involved. This accounts for some of the variability in the course and severity of the disease. What makes things a little more confusing is that many people without MS have antibodies to myelin proteins in their blood, indicating that this is not dangerous on its own but may become so in people who have a faulty control over the immune system. However, there is still a lack of information in general about the origins of auto-immune disease. It is still thought possible that a virus protein that looks very similar to something in the myelin sheath could be the target of the auto-immune response.

Immunology research has made a lot of progress in finding proteins in myelin and oligodendrocytes that might be responsible for stimulating the immune response. The trick now is to work out which proteins may be involved in individual people with MS. Recent research has suggested that a protein called myelin oligodendrocyte glycoprotein (MOG) could be a major target of the immune response in a proportion of people with MS. If such proteins can be identified, it should be possible to develop treatments that switch the immune cells back into a state in which they recognize the proteins as 'self' once again. Copaxone, a drug that is already licensed for use in MS and reduces the number of relapses in some patients, works by trying to reverse the auto-immunity in a relatively non-specific way. Some early clinical trials of more specific therapies that work in this way have recently taken place. They have not yet been entirely successful and have taught us that there is a lot of variability in the immune response between individuals with MS. Some people gained benefit from the therapies, whereas others were made worse because the immune response to self was increased. Although these early clinical trials have been somewhat disappointing, lessons have been learnt, and improved approaches to turning this research into therapies are being developed. It remains a very important area of research because it should be possible to switch off this immune attack against self and thereby completely stop the effects of MS in a specific way without disturbing the parts of the immune system that we need to fight infection.

It needs to be pointed out here that there is actually no general agreement in the scientific community that MS really is an auto-immune disease. Indeed, some other degenerative process within the cells of the brain and spinal cord may stimulate inflammation in the central nervous system, a topic explored later in this chapter.

HOW DO IMMUNE CELLS GET ACROSS THE BLOOD-BRAIN BARRIER?

Whether MS is an auto-immune disease or not becomes a less critical concern if it is possible to stop the immune response at other levels. One of the most promising approaches to new therapies has been to try to stop the immune cells entering into the nervous system from the blood. Immune cells that are looking for their antigen stick to certain blood-vessel walls using sticky molecules called 'cell adhesion molecules'. Immunology research has identified a large number of these molecules, and we now know which ones are very important for sticking T-lymphocytes to blood-vessel walls in MS. Precisely where these sticky molecules are turned on in the blood vessels that supply the brain with oxygen probably determines where a new MS lesion will occur, but this is not yet known for certain. This fundamental research has now been developed into one of the latest therapies to be tested for MS treatment. The drug is called Tysabri (previously known as Antegren or Natalizumab) and is an antibody that sits on the cell adhesion molecule and stops the

T-lymphocyte sticking to the blood vessel. T-lymphocytes unable to stick to the blood-vessel wall cannot enter into the nervous system to cause inflammation. The clinical benefits that this new drug might bring are detailed in the previous chapter (see page 195).

Research into how cells of the immune system actually recognize antigens and then turn on the inflammatory response is also a fruitful area in developing new therapies. For an immune response to be kicked off, cells within the affected tissue (in this case the brain and spinal cord) must show the T-lymphocytes the 'foreign' antigen so that the T-lymphocytes know that they are in the right place and must now do their job. This is done through a complicated lock and key system. Several keys must be put into their respective locks in the right order for the T-lymphocyte to be turned on. This is obviously a great opportunity for developing drugs that block either the locks or the keys, and many experimental therapies are being developed to do this. Statins, the well-known drugs developed to lower cholesterol levels in the blood, have been shown to interfere in this mechanism and are now being tested in clinical trials as a therapy for MS.

Immunology research has also told us a lot about how the immune cells move through the blood-vessel walls and then, once in the central nervous system, how they work to attract other immune cells and multiply to produce the characteristic area of inflammation visible on an MRI scan. These steps are of course more complicated than they sound, involving a family of molecules called 'cytokines', each of which plays a defined role in the immune response. A sub-family of the cytokines, called 'chemokines', is involved in attracting more immune cells to an area of inflammation. Cytokines have an intricate regulatory/modulating interaction with immune cells. It seems that they can either assist in the destructive immune response against myelin by helping to maintain the inflammation that precedes demyelination, or do quite the opposite and turn the immune response into one that supports repair and recovery. If the messages that cytokines bring can be manipulated, it may be possible to turn off the aggressive attack and stop the auto-immune response. Immunology researchers are still discovering new cytokines and studying how they work in the intricate network of molecules and cells that consti-tutes the immune response. This fundamental research helps us understand how we fight off infection, but MS researchers in particular have made great progress in understanding how parts of the cytokine network can be manipulated to turn off MS-like disease in animal models. However, one complication has been that many of these cytokines work together to produce an end result, so stop-ping just one of them acting may have little effect on the disease. In addition, some of these molecules can be involved in amplifying the immune response at the begin-ning, then also play a role in stimulating repair processes. Therefore, stopping them working could have both good and bad effects because we know that some MS lesions are in the damage stage whilst others are in the repair stage. Nevertheless, many early stage clinical trials of new experimental drugs, either alone or in combination with others, have been designed either to stop certain cytokines working, or to mimic the effect of the ones that shut down the immune response and stimulate repair. Most of these experimental therapies are at very early stages, but they have arisen from fundamental MS research into how the immune system damages myelin.

WHY DOES THE IMMUNE ATTACK KEEP COMING BACK?

Some other auto-immune diseases result in relapsing inflammatory attacks to the target tissues rather than a sustained attack. A sustained attack might well prove fatal in some of these conditions, whereas a time-restricted relapse allows the body's own repair systems to be activated. This is one of the great mysteries of MS. When a relapse occurs it is due to the rapid entry of immune cells into the nervous system. Yet, as described earlier, the immune system of most people with MS can eventually turn this off and a period of remission follows. The question is, why does it happen again and again, or why for some people does it never happen again, leaving them free from the effects of MS for the rest of their lives?

There have been many suggestions over the years about what precipitates an attack, some of which sound believable and others unlikely. Studies have been made into the effects of infection, stress and trauma on MS. It is popularly believed that surgery and head injuries may accelerate the development of MS, as may stressful life events, such as divorce, unemployment or moving house. A study that threw doubt on these factors precipitating MS did reveal an increase in respiratory, gastrointestinal and skin infections in the two weeks before an MS attack. There is still a general feeling among medical professionals that many different viral infections can trigger attacks of MS, but real scientific evidence is lacking. Clearly research that provides information such as this may ultimately help in the management of MS. However, it is difficult to think of a trigger that would cause one person to have as many as four or five attacks in a year, and another person to have only one in several years. This is definitely an area of MS that requires more research.

What causes demyelination in MS?

One thing researchers are certain about is that oligodendrocytes and myelin are destroyed by the inflammatory process that occurs during a relapse. The damage is likely to have been brought about via several different routes, but all related to the inflammation. First, T-lymphocytes may directly attack oligodendrocytes, which then leads to destruction of the myelin sheath. Second, antibodies produced by B-lymphocytes attach to myelin and the oligodendrocytes, which are then killed. Third, substances released by the immune cells that are meant to kill bacteria are known to be toxic to oligodendrocytes and neurons. Thus, there is a combination of a targeted attack by immune cells and a more non-specific release of toxic chemicals, both of which contribute to demyelination.

CAN THE MYELIN DAMAGE BE STOPPED?

In order to stop the damage described above, there are two main options. Either the immune cells must be stopped at a much earlier stage before they have a chance to cause the damage, or the toxic chemicals and antibodies must be blocked or removed. Blocking the antibodies can be compared to putting some Blu-Tack into a keyhole to stop insertion of the key, while removing toxic chemicals is a bit like mopping up industrial spills with something that neutralizes the chemical, albeit on a much smaller scale. Some of the toxic chemicals that immune cells produce to kill other cells are now known, and researchers are studying ways in which their effects can be stopped. So far it has been possible to protect oligodendrocytes and myelin against this toxic attack when studying cells in a dish (cell culture) and also in animal models that mimic MS. A family of proteins called 'survival factors' can help oligodendrocytes defend themselves from this attack by protecting them from dying. It is also possible to mop up some of the toxic chemicals using a new group of potential drugs called 'free radical scavengers'. These approaches to developing new therapies have yet to be translated into clinical trials, but some early trials are at the initial planning stages.

When damaging antibodies that are produced by B-lymphocytes stick to oligodendrocytes or myelin, they punch holes in the outside of the cells by bringing in another family of proteins called 'complement proteins'. These proteins literally make a hole in the cell and then, of course, the cell dies. All the broken pieces of myelin are then gathered up by the rubbish disposal agents, called 'macrophages'. Research has revealed that it is possible to stop the complement proteins from working using a natural 'complement inhibitor' that is found in the body. So far this promising approach for developing new treatments has been successful in animals, but has yet to be tried in people. Rather than stopping the damaging antibodies from working, would it be possible to remove the cells – the B-lymphocytes – that make the antibodies? A phase two clinical trial is already under way with a drug called Rituximab to see if this approach benefits people with MS.

DOES REMYELINATION OCCUR NATURALLY?

Once myelin sheaths around nerve fibres are destroyed, their rapid replacement is vital for two reasons. First, we need to replace the myelin so that fast electrical signals blocked by demyelination can be restored along with normal neurological function. Second, covering the bare nerve fibre with a thick myelin sheath once again protects it from further damage by the immune cells. Research using post-mortem tissue from MS brains has revealed that this repair process happens naturally during the early years of MS, and may even continue in some people for a lot longer. As with many other aspects of MS, the success of remyelination can vary markedly from one person to another. One can speculate that if remyelination is totally successful after the first few attacks, and the person then has no further attacks, the central nervous system will have been restored to normal and will be free from MS.

WHY DOES REMYELINATION EVENTUALLY FAIL IN MS?

When a neuropathologist examines a brain at autopsy that has been affected by MS, the one thing immediately evident is the sclerotic plaque (scar tissue). The fact that this can be seen reveals that the repair process has failed. We do not know at what stage it fails because we do not yet have MRI measures that can follow the history of remyelination in the living brain. But fail it does at some stage. Why it fails is one of the unanswered questions of MS research. One possibility for the failure is thought to be a lack of 'oligodendrocyte progenitor cells', which can make new oligodendrocytes. Perhaps they are all destroyed by the repeated attacks of inflammation. However, several research laboratories have used MS tissues to show that this is not true. It is now thought more likely that the cells are somehow prevented from doing their job. Either they are stopped from working correctly by the presence of the wrong signals in the damaged area, or because the nerve fibres have also been damaged by the inflammation and are now not healthy enough to have myelin wrapped around them. Some of the signals that tell oligodendrocytes to wrap around the nerve fibres to produce myelin have recently been found.

CAN MYELIN REPAIR BE STIMULATED?

Just as the process of inflammation involves many different chemical signals working at the same time, so does the repair process. It has been a painstaking task over many years to work out what signals lead to effective repair, but research has succeeded in identifying many of them. Now it is a matter of working out which ones are missing or changed in the non-repairing MS lesion. If the missing signals can be discovered, it will be possible to design therapies to replace them. An alternative to encouraging or switching the natural repair process back on would be to put new cells back in by a process called 'transplantation'. A lot of recent research has looked at the best type of cells for transplantation, an approach that has proven very successful in animal studies. The main obstacles to this working in people with MS are calculating how to get enough human cells to put into the areas of damage, and how to get them to go to all the many areas of damage. Significant progress is being made in this area of research, with the first clinical trials currently being planned for transplanting cells to make new oligodendrocytes.

DOES THE BRAIN ADAPT TO THE DAMAGE?

As a child, you may well have been told that you did not use enough of your brain at school. It is indeed true that we have a degree of spare capacity. The very fact that we can learn new skills at any age tells us that the brain does not have fixed circuits like a computer, but can change to accept new challenges. The damage that MS causes to the brain and spinal cord circuits presents some very real and new challenges. If one part of the brain is damaged, can another part take over from it? This is probably something that goes on without our knowing. Research using a relatively new brain-scanning method, called 'functional MRI', has shown that the brain affected by MS is capable of adapting to meet the new challenges. It is now important to work out ways to make this process even more effective.

Why does MS become progressive at later stages?

Very early studies on MS showed that, in addition to the myelin sheath, the actual nerve fibre itself, the axon, could be damaged by the inflammatory process. However, it has only recently been recognized that a build-up of damage to an increasing number of axons following repeated attacks of MS is very likely to be responsible for the progressive nature of MS. This means that when MS enters the secondary progressive phase, the build-up of symptoms is mainly caused by the loss of axons and the neurons that produce them, rather than the attacks of inflammation. At later stages of MS, this process of axon loss appears to continue in the absence of inflammation. The loss of the nerve cells, or neurons, is called 'neurodegeneration', and is something that also occurs in other conditions affecting the nervous system, such as Alzheimer's and Parkinson's disease.

WHAT TRIGGERS AXON LOSS?

It is thought to be the intensity of the inflammation that occurs during MS attacks that determines whether the axons are just temporarily incapacitated or are permanently and irreversibly damaged. Our knowledge of what actually causes both the temporary and permanent damage to the axons is relatively poor, and is a new area of research. This injury to axons probably starts early on, but becomes noticeable as symptoms only when all the spare capacity is used up. When oligodendrocytes and myelin sheaths are destroyed by immune cells it is thought that the axons are literally caught up in the crossfire and are damaged in a non-specific way. More recent research has also shown that when axons are stripped of their myelin sheaths they try to work even harder than previously. This can result in their effectively killing themselves.

CAN NEURONS BE PROTECTED?

One very important aspect of developing new treatments for MS must be to discover new ways of protecting axons and neurons from dying. This is called 'neuroprotection'. The theory is that if neuroprotective therapies could be started early enough, MS would not enter a secondary progressive phase. If combined with treatments described earlier that stop the inflammation, the damage to the nervous system caused by MS should be stopped completely. Although this is a relatively new area of drug development for MS, researchers are learning from previous research on other conditions in which neurons die, such as Parkinson's disease and motor neurone disease. Pharmaceutical companies that are developing new drugs to slow down or stop these conditions are now planning to carry out clinical trials of the same drugs for MS. This is already proving promising in the laboratory, and a number of neuroprotective treatment approaches should soon be in early clinical trials.

Hope for the future

The previous sections have described briefly some of the work that is ongoing in many different areas of MS research. Compared with a decade ago there has been a substantial increase in the volume of research being conducted. The research is funded primarily by both medical charities and government agencies, often in partnership. MS societies round the world also contribute to a host of research projects specific to the disease in a search for its cause, viable treatments, better diagnosis and eventual cure. When you look at their expenditure, the National MS Society of the USA funds about three-quarters of the total, while 40 per cent of the projects supported by European MS societies are funded by the MS Society of Great Britain and Northern Ireland. More recently the pharmaceutical industry has become interested in the area of MS therapeutics and is beginning to cooperate with the charities and agencies to fund important research.

At the end of 2004 there were 135 clinical trials ongoing around the world of over 70 different drugs for the treatment of MS. Of these trials 108 represent trials of disease modifying therapies and, although many of these therapies will not make it into the neurologist's armoury, some are very promising. This must be viewed against the situation 20 years ago when there were only a handful of agents available for testing in clinical trials. There has never before been so much promise for new treatments for MS that have been based on fundamental research on the disease mechanisms that underlie this enigmatic and often severely disabling disease. Although we still await the arrival of a drug, or combination of drugs, that really stops the onslaught of MS on the nervous system, there is good reason to be hopeful.

Useful Addresses

Organizations specializing in MS

The Multiple Sclerosis Society
MS National Centre
372 Edgware Road, London NW2 6ND
Tel: 020 8438 0700
Fax: 020 8438 0701
Freephone helpline: 0808 800 8000 (weekdays 9am to 9pm)
E-mail: info@mssociety.org.uk
Website: www.mssociety.org.uk

MS Society, Scotland
National Office, Ratho Park, 88 Glasgow Road, Ratho Station,
Edinburgh EH28 8PP
Tel: 0131 335 4050
Fax: 0131 335 4051
E-mail: admin@mssocietyscotland.org.uk
Website: www.mssocietyscotland.org.uk

MS Society, Northern Ireland
34 Annadale Avenue, Belfast BT7 3JJ
Tel: 02890 802 802
Fax: 02890 802 803

The MS Society offers advice and an information service by letter and phone (9am to 5pm). Its Helpline is staffed by advice workers offering an information service on MS. The MS Society also provides a network of over 350 local branches. It is the largest provider of funds for research into MS in the United Kingdom, these being administered through a medical research advisory committee. It also operates respite care centres, and publishes *MS Matters* (six times a year), and a range of information publications free. It is a member of the Multiple Sclerosis International Federation (MSIF).

The Multiple Sclerosis Society of Ireland
Dartmouth House, Grand Parade, Dublin 6, Ireland
Tel: (01) 269 4599
Fax: (01) 269 3746
Helpline: 1850 233 233
E-mail: info@ms-society.ie
Website: www.ms-society.ie

The MS Society of Ireland aims to 'enable and empower people with MS to live the life of their choice to their fullest potential'. It provides a countrywide network of local branches and counsellors, funds specialised community workers and runs a telephone advice and counselling line. Publications include an information pack on all aspects of MS. It is also a member of the Multiple Sclerosis International Federation.

Multiple Sclerosis International Federation (MSIF)
Skyline House, 3rd Floor, 200 Union Street, London SE1 0LX
Tel: 020 7620 1911
Fax: 020 7620 1922
E-mail: info@msif.org
Website: www.msif.org

MSIF, established in 1967, operates a global network invested in wanting to 'eliminate MS and its devastating effects'. Check for the latest information on MS through its website and publications: *MS in Focus* and *MS Guide: Treatment and Management*. It also supports new and existing MS societies and creates forums for international research, debate and developing good practice, such as improving the quality of life for all people with MS around the world. Its Sylvia Lawry Centre for Multiple Sclerosis Research in Munich has the world's largest MS database collected from 43 clinical trials and natural history studies, adding up to 62,000 patient years.

MS Decisions
Website: www.msdecisions.org.uk

An independent website funded by the NHS specifically to help people with MS to decide whether or not to begin disease modifying drug therapy.

The Multiple Sclerosis Research Trust
Spirella Building, Bridge Road, Letchworth, Herts SG6 4ET
Tel: 01462 476 700
Fax: 01462 476 710
E-mail: info@mstrust.org.uk
Website: www.mstrust.org.uk

The MS Trust is a very good source of information about MS, funds applied research and works closely with MS nurses. In particular, it promotes positive approaches to managing MS through information and education.

Multiple Sclerosis Resource Centre
7 Peartree Business Centre, Peartree Road, Stanway, Colchester, Essex CO3 0JN
Tel: 01206 505 444
24-hour counselling line: 0800 783 0518
Website: www.msrc.co.uk

The MS Resource Centre offers advice on all aspects of living with MS day to day. Its magazine *New Pathways* and an information pack are available on request.

Multiple Sclerosis National Therapy Centres
Bradbury House, 155 Barkers Lane, Bedford MK41 9RX
Tel: 01231 325 781
Fax: 01234 365 242
E-mail: info@ms-selfhelp.org
Website: www.ms-selfhelp.org

Many excellent MS therapy centres operate throughout Great Britain and Northern Ireland offering information, advice and practical help. They provide a wide range of therapies for managing MS, which include physiotherapy, yoga, speech therapy, chiropody, diet control, continence advice, reflexology, aromatherapy and counselling. Some centres also operate their own hyperbaric oxygen treatment chambers.

The UK Multiple Sclerosis Tissue Bank
Division of Neuroscience and Psychological Medicine, Imperial College Faculty of Medicine, Charing Cross Campus, Fulham Palace Road, London W6 8RF
Tel: 020 8846 7324
Fax: 020 8846 7500
E-mail: ukmstissuebank@imperial.ac.uk
Website: www.ukmstissuebank.imperial.ac.uk

Based at Charing Cross Hospital, the Tissue Bank coordinates the donation and collection of MS brain and spinal cord from people who have MS, and those who don't, who are happy to give consent while they are alive for their tissues to be used for MS research after they die. The Bank then distributes tissue to vital research projects worldwide.

National MS Society (USA)
Website: www.nmss.org

The MS Awareness Foundation (USA)
Website: www.msawareness.org

Multiple Sclerosis Australia (MSA)
Studdy MS Center, Joseph Street, Lidcombe NSW 2141
Tel: (61) 02 9640 0600
E-mail: info@mssociety.com.au
Website: www.msaustralia.org.au

Multiple Sclerosis Society of Canada (Société canadienne de la sclérose en plaques)
175 Bloor Street East, Suite 700, North Tower,
Toronto ON M4W 3R8
Tel: (1) 416 922 6065
E-mail: info@mssociety.ca
Website: www.mssociety.ca

Cyprus Multiple Sclerosis Association
67-69 Ayiou Nicolaou Street, 2408, Engomi, Nicosia
Tel: (357) 22 590949
E-mail: multips@logos.net.cy

Multiple Sclerosis Society of Malta (MSSM)
PO Box 209, Valetta
Tel: (356) 418 066
E-mail: lagius@onvol.net

MS Society of New Zealand Inc. (MSSNZ)
Level 4, Hallenstein House
276-278 Lambton Quay
PO Box 2627, Wellington
Tel: (64) 4 499 4677
Website: www.msnz.org.nz

Organisations dealing with general disability and caring

AbilityNet
Helpline: 0800 269 545 (weekdays 9am to 5pm)
Website: www.abilitynet.org.uk

Specialises in providing information and assessments for computer equipment. It can also assist with installation, training and support.

Advisory, Conciliation and Arbitration Service (ACAS)
Brandon House, 180 Borough High Street, London SE1 1LW
Helpline: 08457 474 747 (weekdays 8am to 6pm)
Textphone: 08456 061 600 (weekdays 8am to 6pm)
Website: www.acas.org.uk

Offers expert advice on employment issues, good practice in general and also deals with individual cases.

Association of Crossroads Care Attendant Schemes Ltd
10 Regent Place, Rugby, Warwickshire CV21 2PN
Tel: 0845 450 0350
Fax: 01788 565 498
E-mail: communications@crossroads.org.uk
Website: www.crossroads.org.uk

Crossroads promotes, supports and delivers a high quality service that aims to relieve stress for carers and people with care needs by offering domiciliary support locally.

Automobile Association (AA)
Freephone: 0800 262 050

BBC Helpline
Tel: 0800 044 044

British Acupuncture Council
63 Jeddo Road, London W12 9HQ
Tel: 020 8735 0400
Fax: 020 8735 0404
E-mail: info@acupuncture.org.uk
Website: www.acupuncture.org.uk

British Association for Counselling and Psychotherapy (BACP)
BACP House, 35-37 Albert Street, Rugby, Warwickshire CV21 2SG
Tel: 0870 443 5252
Website: www.bacp.co.uk

For details of accredited counsellors, psychologists and therapists.

British Medical Acupuncture Society
BMAS House, 3 Winnington Court, Northwich, Cheshire CW8 1AQ
Tel: 01606 786 782
Fax: 01606 786 783
E-mail: admin@medical-acupuncture.org.uk
Website: www.medical-acupuncture.co.uk

British Red Cross
UK Office, 44 Moorfields, London EC2Y 9AL
Tel: 0870 170 7000
Fax: 020 7562 2000
E-mail: information@redcross.org.uk
Website: www.redcross.org.uk

Carers UK
20–25 Glasshouse Yard, London EC1A 4JT
Tel: 020 7490 8818
Helpline: 0808 808 7777 (Wednesday to Thursday, 10am to 12pm, 2pm to 4pm)
Website: www.carersonline.org.uk

The leading voluntary organisation working to advise all carers and encourage them to recognise their own needs. Carers UK promotes the interests of carers within government and other policy makers, and provides information leaflets and a national helpline run by qualified and trained staff.

Citizens Advice (formerly The National Association of Citizens Advice Bureau)
Myddleton House, 115-123 Pentonville Road, London N1 9LZ
Tel: 020 7833 2181
Website: www.citizensadvice.org.uk or www.adviceguide.org.uk

Source of help with welfare rights, housing and disability advice. Check your phonebook or their website for details of your local Citizens Advice office. They also operate an online advice guide.

The Continence Foundation
Helpline: 0845 345 0165 (weekdays 9:30am to 1pm)
Website: www.continence-foundation.org.uk

For easily available personal and confidential advice on bladder or bowel control problems

Department of Health
Website: www.dh.gov.uk or www.carers.gov.uk

Check its main website for general information on health and social care and details of legislation such as the Carers and Disabled Children Act 2000.

Department for Work and Pensions (DWP)
Disability Unit, Level 6, The Adelphi, 1-11 John Adam Street, London WC2N 6HT
Helpline: 020 7712 2171 (weekdays 9am to 5pm)
Website: www.disability.gov.uk

For in-depth information on disability legislation, policy and public consultations.

Dial UK (National Association of Disablement Information and Advice Lines)
St Catherine's, Tickhill Road, Balby, Doncaster DN4 8QN
Tel: 01302 310 123
Fax: 01302 310 404
E-mail: enquiries@dialuk.org.uk
Website: www.dialuk.info

A national network of disability information and advice services aiming to provide comprehensive and confidential information and an advice service on any matter relating to disability. Contact them for a list of local DIAL groups in England and Wales.

The Disabled Living Foundation
380–384 Harrow Road, London W9 2HU
Helpline: 0845 130 9177
E-mail: advice@dlf.org.uk
Website: www.dlf.org.uk

For information and advice on daily living equipment for people with a disability.

Disability Alliance
Universal House, 88–94 Wentworth Street, London E1 7SA
Tel: 020 7247 8776
Fax: 020 7247 8765
Website: www.disabilityalliance.org

The leading authority on social service benefits for disabled people. It publishes the invaluable *Disability Rights Handbook*.

Disability Law Service (DLS)
39-45 Cavell Street, London E1 2BP

Tel: 020 7791 9800
Fax: 020 7791 9802
Minicom: 020 7791 9801
E-mail: advice@dls.org.uk
Website: www.dls.org.uk

For free and confidential legal advice and representation for people with a disability. The MS Society specifically funds a fast-track service for people with MS, which you can access by saying that you are *contacting the DLS on behalf of the MS Society.*

Disability Rights Commission (DRC)
DRC Helpline, FREEPOST MID 02164, Stratford-upon-Avon CV37 9BR
Helpline: 08457 622 633 (weekdays 8am to 8pm)
Textphone: 08457 622 644
Website: www.drc-gb.org

For specific information about the Disability Discrimination Acts. The DRC gives advice and information to disabled people, employers and service providers.

Dogs for the Disabled
The Frances Hay Centre, Blacklocks Hill, Banbury,
Oxon OX17 2BS
Tel: 01295 252 600
Fax: 01295 252 668
E-mail: info@dogsforthedisabled.org
Website: www.dogsforthedisabled.org

Trains and supplies skilled assistance or companion dogs which perform a wide range of everyday tasks for their owners. They aim to enable disabled adults and children to be independent through partnership and enhance their quality of life.

Drinkline
Tel: 0800 917 8282

Employment Opportunities for People with Disabilities
53 New Broad Street, London EC2M 1SL
Tel: 020 7448 5420
Fax: 020 7374 4913
Minicom: 020 7374 6884
E-mail: info@eopps.org
Website: operations@eopps.org

Employment Opportunities aims through training, preparation and guidance to help people with disabilities find jobs matched to their talents and aspirations by persuading employers to positively recognise abilities and potentials.

InContact
United House, North Road, London N7 9DP
Tel: 0870 770 3246
Fax: 0870 770 3249
Website: www.incontact.org

An organisation for people affected by bowel and bladder problems.

IndependentAge
6 Avonmore Road, London W14 8RL
Tel: 020 7605 4200 or 08457 585 680 to request a copy of the guides
Fax: 020 7605 4201
Website: www.independentage.org.uk

Supports people over the age of forty who are permanently unable to work due to physical disability, as well as enabling older people on low incomes to live independently with dignity and peace of mind. It publishes two very useful guides: *60-Wise* and *60-Wise at Home*.

John Grooms Housing Association
50 Scrutton Street, London EC2A 4XQ
Tel: 020 7452 2000
Website: www.johngrooms.org.uk/housing

King's Fund
11 - 13 Cavendish Square, London W1G 0AN
Tel: 020 7307 2400
Fax: 020 7307 2801
Website: www.kingsfund.org.uk

A policy advisory body and research centre that informs and supports people with different conditions and their carers.

Leonard Cheshire
30 Millbank, London SW1P 4QD
Tel: 020 7802 8200
Fax: 020 7802 8250
E-mail: info@lc-uk.org
Website: www.leonard-cheshire.org

Mobility Advice and Insurance Service (MAVIS)
Crowthorne Business Estate, Old Wokingham Road, Crowthorne, Berkshire RG45 6XD
Tel: 01344 661 000
Website: www.dft.gov.uk/access/mavis

For practical advice on driving, vehicle adaptation and suitable vehicle types for both drivers and passengers. Part of the Department of Transport.

Motability
Website: www.motability.co.uk

Motability Car Scheme
City Gate House, 22 Southwark Bridge Road, London SE1 9HB
Tel: 0845 456 4566

Motability Wheelchair & Scooter Scheme
Newbury Road, Enham Alamein, Andover, Hampshire SP11 6JS
Tel: 01264 384 480

Enables disabled people and their families to become mobile by supplying cars, scooters or wheelchairs.

National Centre for Independent Living
250 Kennington Lane, London SE11 5RD
Tel: 020 7587 1663
Website: www.ncil.org.uk

NHS Direct
Website: www.direct.gov.uk

A clear website that provides public service information on disability, health and well-being, access to health services, employment, independent living and rights.

NHS Smoking Helpline
Tel: 0800 169 0 169

National Institute for Clinical Excellence (NICE)
MidCity Place, 71 High Holborn, London WC1V 6NA
Tel: 020 7067 5800
Fax: 020 7067 5801
E-mail: nice@nice.nhs.uk
Website: www.nice.org.uk

The booklet, *Multiple Sclerosis: Understanding NICE guidance – information for people with multiple sclerosis, their families and carers, and the public* can be ordered from the NHS Response Line on 0870 155 5455 and quote reference number NO367.

The National Institute of Medical Herbalists (NIMH)
Elm House, 54 Mary Arches Street, Exeter EX4 3BA
Tel: 01392 426 022

Fax: 01392 498 963
E-mail: nimh@ukexeter.freeserve.co.uk
Website: www.nimh.org.uk

Pilates Foundation
PO Box 36052, London SW16 1XQ
Tel: 07071 781 859
Fax: 020 8696 0088
Website: www.pilatesfoundation.com

Phab (Physically Handicapped and Able-Bodied)
Summit House, Wandle Road, Croydon CR0 1DF
Tel: 020 8667 9443
Fax: 020 86811399
E-mail: info@phabengland.org.uk
Website: www.phabengland.org.uk

Focuses on integrating able-bodied and disabled people in all aspects of life.

Quitline
Tel: 0800 00 22 00

RADAR (Royal Association for Disability and Rehabilitation)
12 City Forum, 250 City Road, London EC1V 8AF
Tel: 020 7250 3222
Fax: 020 7250 0212
Minicom: 020 7250 4119
E-mail: radar@radar.org.uk
Website: www.radar.org.uk

An umbrella organisation that provides information on access, education, employment, housing, holidays, mobility and benefits. It operates the National Key Scheme that gains users access to locked public toilets suitable for people with disabilities. Renowned for representing the interests of disabled people nationally.

Relate
Tel: 01788 573241
Website: www.relate.org.uk

For advice on relationships. Offers support by phone, through the website or face-to-face, consultations, mediation, relationship counselling, sex therapy and workshops.

Sexual Dysfunction Association
Windmill Place Business Centre, 2-4 Windmill Lane, Southall, Middlesex UB2 4NJ
Helpline: 0870 774 3571
Website: www.sda.uk.net

For men and women who experience sexual dysfunction and their partners.

Skill (National Bureau for Students with Disabilities)
Chapter House, 18-20 Crucifix Lane, London SE1 3JW
Tel/Minicom: 020 7450 0620
Fax: 020 7450 0650
Information Service: 0800 328 5050 or 020 7657 2337 (open Tuesdays 11:30am to 1:30pm and Thursdays 1:30pm to 3:30pm)
E-mail: skill@skill.org.uk
Website: www.skill.org.uk

Promotes opportunities for young people and adults with any kind of disability in post-16 education, training and employment.

Terrence Higgins Trust
52-54 Grays Inn Road, London WC1X 8JU
Tel: 020 7831 0330
Fax: 020 7242 0121
E-mail: info@tht.org.uk
Website: www.tht.org.uk

Tourism for All (formerly Holiday Care)

Tourism for All, The Hawkins Suite, Enham Place, Enham Alamein,
Andover SP11 6JS
Tel: 0845 124 9971
Website: www.tourismforall.info

Offering people with disabilities opportunities for a holiday by
providing information on accommodation, visitor attractions, activity holidays and respite care centres, both in the UK and abroad.

Tripscope

The Vassell Court, Gill Avenue, Bristol BS16 2QQ
Helpline: 08457 585 641 (weekdays 9:30am to 4:30pm)
Website: www.tripscope.org.uk

For travel advice and transport information for people with disabilities and mobility problems.

Vitalise (formerly Winged Fellowship Trust)

12 City Forum, 250 City Road, London EC1V 8AF
Tel: 0845 345 1972
Fax: 0845 345 1978
Website: www.vitalise.org.uk

Yoga for Health Foundation

Ickwell Bury, Biggleswade, Bedfordshire SG18 9EF
Tel: 01767 627 271
Fax: 01767 627 266
E-mail: admin@yogaforhealthfoundation.co.uk
Website: www.yogaforhealthfoundation.co.uk

A residential treatment centre with special weekend courses and
holidays, and a centre to train teachers to work with people with
disabilities, especially those with MS.

Further Reading

Learning to Live with Multiple Sclerosis R. Povey, R. Dowey and G. Prett (Sheldon Press)

Living with MS Elizabeth Forsythe, MRCS LRCP DPH (Faber and Faber)

McAlpine's Multiple Sclerosis Edited by W. B. Matthews (Longman Group UK Ltd)

Managing the Symptoms of Multiple Sclerosis Randall T. Schapiro (Demos Medical Publishing Inc)

Managing your MS Professor Ian Robinson and Dr Frank Clifford Rose (Class Publishing)

Multiple Sclerosis: A Guide for the Newly-Diagnosed Nancy J Holland et al (Demos Medical Publishing Inc)

Multiple Sclerosis – A Personal Exploration Alexander Burnfield (Souvenir Press)

Multiple Sclerosis – A Self-Help Guide to its Management Judy Graham (HarperCollins)

Multiple Sclerosis – Exploring Sickness and Health Elizabeth Forsythe, MRCS LRCP DPH (Faber and Faber)

Multiple Sclerosis – The Facts W. B. Matthews, DM FRCP (Oxford University Press)

Multiple Sclerosis and Having a Baby: Everything You

needed to Know About Conception, Pregnancy and Parenthood Judy Graham (Healing Arts Press)

Need to Know: Multiple Sclerosis Alexander Burnfield (Heinemann Library)

Standing in the Sunshine: The Story of the MS Breakthrough Cari Loder (Century Press)

Symptom Management in Multiple Sclerosis Randall Schapiro (Costello)

The First Year: Multiple Sclerosis Margaret Blackstone (Constable & Robinson)

The Multiple Sclerosis Fact Book Richard Lechtenberg (F. A. Davis)

Therapeutic Claims in Multiple Sclerosis William Sibley (Demos Medical Publishing Inc)

You and Caring – An Action Plan for Caring at Home Penny Mares (Kings Fund Centre)

Index